ATI TEAS 7TH EDITION 2024 – 2025 STUDY GUIDE

Comprehensive Exam Simulations And In-Depth Answer Explanations | Quick And Easy Exam Prep

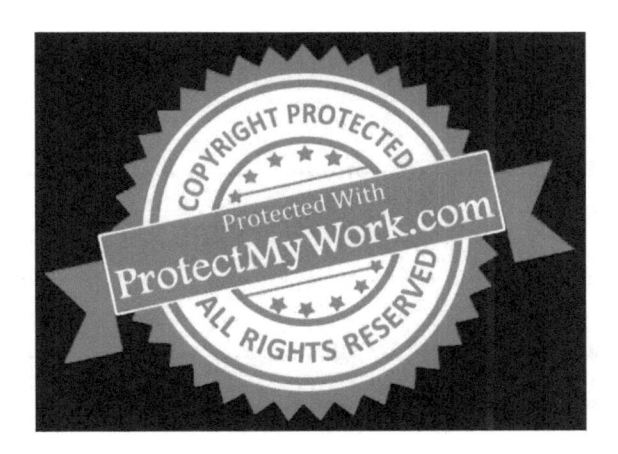

All Rights Reserved.
COPYRIGHT REFERENCE NUMBER: 20556030923S028

BY

Noah Scott

TABLE OF CONTENTS

INTRODUCTION 4

CHAPTER 1: The Reading 6
   Questions and Answers 9

CHAPTER 2: Mathematics 33
   How to prepare for the math test: 33
   Numbers and operations: 34
   Data interpretation: 34
   Test Format: 35
   How to Prepare for the Mathematics Section: 35
   Measurement and data: 36
   Geometry: 37
   Questions & Answers 37

CHAPTER 3: The Science 49
   Body systems: 49
   Question &Answers 53

CHAPTER 4: English and Language Usage 67
   Questions & Answers 69

CHAPTER 5: Reading 82
   Benefits of reading: 82
   Is reading really tiring? 82
   Technology and reading 83
   Preparing for the exam 83

Test Simulation 1 85

Test Simulation 2 112

CONCLUSION 113

INTRODUCTION

A significant number of nursing schools and allied health programs in the United States employ the ATI TEAS, also known as the Test of Essential Academic Skills, as a required admissions test. The ATI TEAS, which was formerly known as the TEAS V, is a test that evaluates a student's intellectual preparedness for the rigorous nature of nursing and other subjects connected to healthcare. Reading, mathematics, science, and proper English and language usage are the four primary subject areas that will be tested on this examination to determine whether or not candidates possess the necessary academic skills. It is a computer-based test with multiple-choice questions, and the timing for each segment is kept distinct.

Structure of the ATI TEAS Exam:

The ATI TEAS exam consists of four sections, with each section containing a specific number of questions and allocated time. The sections are as follows:

1. **Reading (Reading Comprehension):** This section assesses the test-taker's ability to comprehend written information. It typically consists of around 53 questions and has a time limit of 64 minutes.

2. **Mathematics:** The Mathematics section evaluates the student's mathematical skills and knowledge. It usually includes approximately 36 questions to be completed within 54 minutes.

3. **Science:** In this section, the test-taker's understanding of scientific concepts is tested. It comprises about 53 questions and has a time limit of 63 minutes.

4. **English and Language Usage:** This section examines the student's proficiency in English grammar, vocabulary, and language usage. It typically contains around 28 questions and has a time limit of 28 minutes.

Strategies for Dealing with the ATI TEAS Exam:

Preparing for the ATI TEAS exam requires a strategic approach to maximize your performance. Here are some effective strategies to deal with the exam:

1. **Understand the Content:** Review the content areas covered in the exam thoroughly. Familiarize yourself with the types of questions asked in each section and focus on the topics you find most challenging.

2. **Create a Study Plan:** Develop a study plan that allocates sufficient time for each section. Be consistent with your study schedule and set achievable goals to track your progress.

3. **Practice with Sample Questions:** Utilize official ATI TEAS study materials and practice tests to become familiar with the exam format and question types. This will help you build confidence and improve your speed and accuracy.

4. **Focus on Weak Areas:** Identify your weak areas and concentrate on improving them. Allocate more study time to topics where you need improvement.

5. **Time Management:** During the actual exam, manage your time wisely. Work on questions you are confident about first, and then return to more challenging ones later. Avoid spending too much time on a single question.

6. **Elimination Strategy:** If you encounter a challenging question, use the process of elimination to rule out obviously incorrect answers. This increases your chances of selecting the correct option.

7. **Stay Calm and Confident:** Anxiety can negatively impact your performance. Stay calm, focused, and confident during the exam. Remember that adequate preparation increases your chances of success.

8. **Review and Check:** If time permits, review your answers before submitting the exam. Ensure that you have answered all questions and haven't made any careless mistakes.

9. **Get Adequate Rest:** Ensure you get enough rest the night before the exam. Being well-rested can help improve your concentration and cognitive performance during the test.

10. **Test-Taking Strategies:** Familiarize yourself with general test-taking strategies, such as budgeting time, reading instructions carefully, and avoiding random guessing (as there is no penalty for incorrect answers).

By following these strategies and dedicating sufficient time to preparation, you can increase your chances of performing well on the ATI TEAS exam and gain admission to the nursing or healthcare program of your choice.

CHAPTER 1: The Reading

The ATI (Assessment Technologies Institute) exams are used in various nursing and allied health programs to assess students' readiness for the healthcare profession. The reading sections in ATI exams are designed to evaluate a student's ability to comprehend and analyze written information, which is crucial for success in healthcare education and practice. Let's delve into the duration, difficulty, tips to pass, and key aspects of the reading section in ATI exams:

1. DURATION AND DIFFICULTY OF THE ATI READING TEST:

    - Duration: The duration of the reading section in ATI exams may vary depending on the specific exam and the number of questions. Typically, students are given a set amount of time, such as 60 to 90 minutes, to complete the reading section.

    - Difficulty Level: The difficulty level of the ATI reading test can be challenging for some students. The passages may cover a wide range of healthcare-related topics, including medical terminology, patient care scenarios, and healthcare ethics. The questions may involve critical thinking and application of knowledge to real-world situations.

2. HOW TO PASS THE ATI READING TEST:

    - Develop Active Reading Strategies: Engage actively with the passages by underlining or highlighting key information, making notes in the margins, and summarizing the main ideas. This approach will help you retain information and refer back to the text while answering questions.

    - Practice Time Management: Since time is limited during the exam, practice answering reading comprehension questions under timed conditions. This will help you become more efficient in reading and answering questions within the given time frame.

    - Focus on Medical Terminology: Familiarize yourself with medical terminology commonly used in healthcare settings. Understanding these terms will help you comprehend passages related to patient care and medical procedures.

    - Improve Critical Thinking Skills: ATI exams often include questions that require critical thinking and problem-solving abilities. Practice analyzing complex scenarios and making well-reasoned decisions based on the information provided in the passages.

- Review Test-Taking Strategies: Learn and apply test-taking strategies, such as eliminating obviously incorrect options, rephrasing questions to better understand them, and carefully reviewing your answers before submitting.

3. KEY IDEAS AND DETAILS: The ATI reading section may assess your ability to grasp key ideas and details from the provided passages. Here are some key aspects the test may focus on:

- Main Idea: Identify the central theme or purpose of the passage.

- Supporting Details: Comprehend specific information, examples, or evidence provided by the author to support their main idea or argument.

- Inference: Draw logical conclusions based on the information presented in the passage, even if it is not explicitly stated.

- Vocabulary in Context: Understand the meaning of words or phrases based on how they are used in the context of the passage.

- Understanding Patient Scenarios: Analyze patient care scenarios and demonstrate the ability to apply medical knowledge to solve problems and make appropriate decisions.

CRAFT:

In the context of the ATI exam, "craft" refers to the way in which an author constructs and presents a written passage. Understanding an author's craft is essential for comprehending complex texts and analyzing the effectiveness of the writing. The ATI exam may assess your ability to identify various elements of craft, such as:

- **Author's Tone and Style:** Analyzing the author's tone (the author's attitude towards the subject matter) and style (the way the author writes) can provide insights into the intended message and overall impact of the passage.

- **Figurative Language:** Recognizing and interpreting figurative language, such as metaphors, similes, and symbolism, can deepen your understanding of the text and its underlying meaning.

- **Language Features:** Paying attention to literary devices, rhetoric, and persuasive techniques employed by the author can help you identify the author's intent and message.

- **Text Structure:** Understanding how the passage is organized (e.g., cause and effect, problem-solution, chronological order) helps you follow the flow of information and identify key points.

STRUCTURE:

The structure of a passage refers to its organization and the way the content is presented. In the ATI exam, you may encounter passages with different structures, and understanding these structures is crucial for effectively analyzing and answering questions. Common text structures include:

- **Chronological Order:** Information is presented in a time-based sequence, often used in historical or biographical texts.
- **Cause and Effect:** The author explains how certain events or actions lead to specific outcomes.
- **Compare and Contrast:** Differentiates between two or more subjects, highlighting their similarities and differences.
- **Problem-Solution:** The author presents a problem and then proposes one or more solutions.
- **Description:** Provides detailed sensory information about a subject to create a vivid mental image for the reader.
- **Argumentative:** The author presents a clear claim or argument supported by evidence and reasoning.

INTEGRATION OF KNOWLEDGE AND IDEAS: The "Integration of Knowledge and Ideas" is a critical reading skill that involves connecting information from various sources or parts of a text to develop a deeper understanding. In the ATI exam, this skill may be assessed in different ways:

- **Synthesizing Information:** Combining ideas from multiple sources to draw logical conclusions or develop new insights.
- **Evaluating Arguments:** Analyzing the strength and validity of arguments presented in the passage and assessing the credibility of the evidence provided.
- **Making Inferences:** Drawing conclusions based on implicit information, clues, or evidence presented in the text.

- **Comparing and Contrasting:** Identifying similarities and differences between different passages or perspectives on a topic.

- **Identifying Themes:** Recognizing recurring ideas, messages, or lessons in the text.

- **Recognizing Bias:** Being able to identify any bias or subjective viewpoints in the writing and evaluating how it affects the author's message.

Strengthening your reading and critical thinking skills, along with familiarity with healthcare-related topics and medical terminology, will significantly improve your performance in the ATI reading section. Additionally, practice with sample ATI exams and seek study resources to prepare effectively for the reading component of the ATI exam.

To excel in the ATI exam's "Craft and Structure" and "Integration of Knowledge and Ideas" sections, practice analyzing various types of passages, identifying literary devices, and honing your ability to connect information across different sources. Additionally, read widely and critically to enhance your comprehension and analytical skills.

Questions and Answers

The reading that follows will serve as your basis for Questions 1 and 2.

Are you trying to figure out how you can give back to your community, but you can't seem to get beyond a certain roadblock? One of the best investments you can make in the future of your community is to contribute to the enhancement of the educational opportunities available to our youngsters. Even highly qualified educators are feeling the strain to aid students because of inadequate funding for the nation's institutions. With the help of our group-funding programs, you can search through the thousands of instructor programs that are looking for financial support online. These programs were developed by educators who were aware of the requirements necessary to support the achievement of their students. It is not often that you will have the opportunity to donate while simultaneously being aware of the precise destination of that contribution. Make an immediate contribution to help impact the lives of a group of students who reside in your immediate area.

1. Which of the following aspects of this strategy for group finance is not like any of the others?

   A. The contribution is eligible for a tax deduction.

   B. The recipients of your generosity will benefit.

   C. You can trace the movement of your money at any time.

   D. You can assist in the training of new instructors.

   Answer You can always monitor the location of your money.

2. Which of the following describes the word "beset" in the passage, according to the context?

   A. to feel overburdened and worried

   B. to succeed despite challenges

   C. To battle for what you require

   D. to give up in the face of overwhelming challenges

Answer: to feel overburdened and worried

Questions 3–4 are based on the following passage.

   Sonja,

In my opinion, we ought to launch operations most likely in a new place. We have been discussing carrying it out for a very long time, and if we continue to put it off for any longer, there is a possibility that we will never actually get around to executing it. I understand this is a risky move; but I believe that taking some calculated risks is the best way for our business to grow. Consumers in Springdale would really appreciate having one of our stores in their mall, according to the data collected in our focus groups, and business has never been better than it is right now. If we are successful in putting this plan into action, within the next three years we will be able to more than quadruple our current level of profitability. Give me your opinion on the matter.

Thanks,

Gabriela

PS: To make the most of the attention that will be coming our way, we could even announce the expansion after that puff piece on Channel 4 has aired!

3. Which of the following best sums up Sonja and Gabriela's relationship, according to the memo's tone?

    A. Sonja's superior is Gabriela.

    B. Gabriela's superior is Sonja

    C. Gabriela and Sonja are coworkers in the human resources division.

    D. Gabriela and Sonja jointly handle the firm.

Answer: Gabriela and Sonja jointly handle the firm.

4. Which of the following sums up the author's intentions the best?

    A. Open a second site to help an unsuccessful company get back on its feet.

    B. Expand a flourishing company by adding a second site.

    C. Make herself seem to be a stronger leader than Gabriela.

    D. Persuade a coworker to conduct additional study on potential locations for a second site.

Answer: Expand a flourishing company by adding a second site.

Questions 5–7 are based on the following passage.

Teachers all throughout the United States are coming to the realization that there is a significant educational benefit to using film in today's classrooms. It is no longer the goal of showing a movie to pupils while the instructor is working at their desk for them to relax and unwind while watching the film. Films are a versatile medium that can function as a student's textbook, a piece of literature, or an artistic work while also providing them with a new viewpoint on the subject matter that they are studying. The educators who are spearheading this movement understand in order to teach a movie in an effective manner, they will need to spend the same amount of time and effort organizing lessons as they would on any other day. Since this is a class that is learning about World War II, the teacher might easily dim the lights and show the first twenty minutes of "Saving Private Ryan," which was directed by Steven Spielberg. Alternately, the instructor might have the class spend a period of class time dissecting the scene and discussing how Spielberg uses conflict and anxiety to make the spectator care about characters they haven't even met yet.

5. Which of the following best sums up the author's position on the use of film in the classroom?

    A. Young educators who show movies to their students are failing them.

    B. More instructors ought to display "Saving Private Ryan" at its opening sequence during class.

    C. If used properly in the classroom, movies can be excellent teaching tools.

    D. For students who struggle with reading, movies are an effective teaching tool.

Answer: If used properly in the classroom, movies can be excellent teaching tools.

6. Which of the following statements best illustrates how "Saving Private Ryan" may be applied in the classroom?

    A. The ability to evaluate a movie in this way can assist students not only acquire more from their viewing but also develop their critical thinking abilities.

    B. It's not a good idea to show "Saving Private Ryan" in class and then have students work on other projects in the back of the room.

    C. But far too many educators are hesitant to change and are set in their ways.

    D. Another excellent movie that a teacher may show in the classroom is "Jaws."

Answer: The ability to evaluate a movie in this way can assist students not only acquire more from their viewing but also develop their critical thinking abilities.

Passage

    Teachers all throughout the United States are coming to the realization that there is a significant educational benefit to using film in today's classrooms. It is no longer the goal of showing a movie to pupils while the instructor is working at their desk for them to relax and unwind while watching the film. Films are a versatile medium that can function as a student's textbook, a piece of literature, or an artistic work while also providing them with a new viewpoint on the subject matter that they are studying. The educators who are spearheading this movement are well aware that in order to teach a movie in an effective manner, they will need to spend the same amount of time and effort organizing lessons as they would on any other day. Because this is a lesson about World War II, the teacher might just dim the lights and play the first twenty minutes of "Saving Private Ryan," which was directed by Steven Spielberg. Alternately, the instructor might have the class spend a period of class time dissecting the scene and discussing how Spielberg uses conflict and anxiety to make the spectator care about characters they haven't even met yet.

7. Which of the following best describes the term "versatile" as it is used in the passage?

    A. anything with a powerful rhythm

    B. Something rooted in reality

    C. Something that is prone to misunderstanding

    D. anything with a wide range of applications

Answer: anything with a wide range of applications

Questions 8–9 are based on the following pie chart.

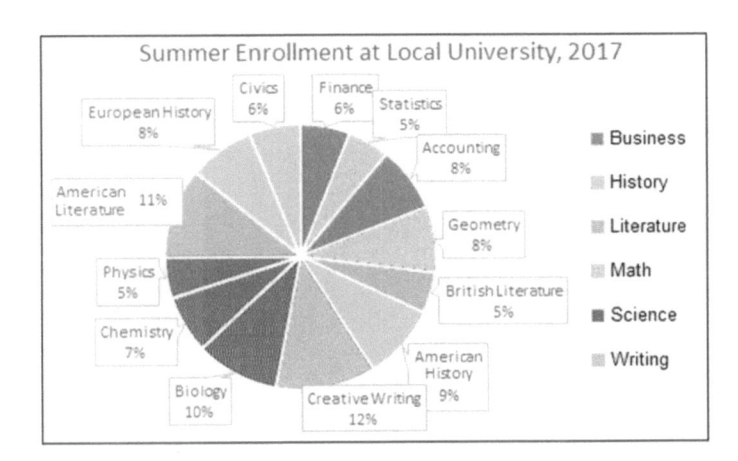

Summer Enrollment at Local University, 2017

- European History 8%
- Civics 6%
- Finance 6%
- Statistics 5%
- Accounting 8%
- American Literature 11%
- Geometry 8%
- Physics 5%
- British Literature 5%
- Chemistry 7%
- American History 9%
- Biology 10%
- Creative Writing 12%

Legend:
- Business
- History
- Literature
- Math
- Science
- Writing

8. Which department in 2017 had the largest enrollment for its summer courses?

   A. Business
   B. History
   C. Literature
   D. Science

Answer: History

9. Which of the following statements about the data in the graph above is true?

   A. The most popular class this summer is American History
   B. This summer, finance is the least popular subject.
   C. The most popular science class is biology.
   D. Most students just enroll in the most crucial classes.

Answer: The most popular science class is biology.

Passage

The first mention of the Terracotta Army in a book about China's first emperor is sought after by the reader. What should he or she search for? The first mention of the Terracotta Army in a book about China's first emperor is sought after by the reader.

10. What should he or she search for?

    A. The glossary
    B. The table of contents
    C. The afterword
    D. The index

Answer: The index

Questions 11 to 13 are based on the following passage.

Hello Karla

Since you have been chosen as Employee of the Year for 2018, please accept our congratulations. We are grateful for the dedication you have shown to our company as well as all of the hard work you have put in. When the committee gathered to assess the prospective award recipients, you were in the lead because of the long hours that you and your team put in, as well as the 11% growth in global sales that your team delivered despite the weakening economy. This honor comes with a brand-new parking spot, an incentive of $5,000, and a plaque that will be placed close to the entrance of our office. This information is common knowledge. Please pay Su Yun a visit as soon as you can so that she can take your official photograph.

I am thankful for everything that you do. Fahmida Bukhari is currently serving in the capacity of director of human resources at Systematic Alliance Reserve, Inc.

11. Which of the following passage's assertions is true?

    A. Global sales increased by 11% under Karla's leadership.

    B. Karla's labour of love is valued by Mrs. Bukhari.

    C. Karla is devoted to Systematic Alliance Reserve, Inc., her employer.

    D. Karla will prefer her new parking spot to her previous one.

Answer: Global sales increased by 11% under Karla's leadership.

12. Which of the following best sums up the author's perspective?

    A. Business is a team sport, thus it's critical to appreciate everyone's contributions to a task.

    B. Giving employees sizable monetary bonuses is the best method to keep them from quitting a company.

    C. People who put in a lot of effort and accomplish in spite of their challenges should be rewarded.

D. Businesses in difficult economic times can only survive by laying off layoffs.

Answer: People who put in a lot of effort and accomplish in spite of their challenges should be rewarded.

Questions 13 to 15 are based on the following passage.

A spacesuit is made up of various components. The astronaut's chest is covered by the Hard Upper Torso. The gloves are attached to the arm assembly, which covers the arms. The astronaut's head is protected by the helmet and Extravehicular Visor Assembly while still allowing for as much vision as feasible.

The legs and feet of the astronaut are protected by the Lower Torso Assembly. The suit's flexible components are constructed from multiple layers of material. The layers provide a variety of purposes, such as preserving oxygen within the spacesuit and shielding against space dust.

Astronauts don a Liquid Cooling and Ventilation Garment underneath their spacesuit. This tight-fitting garment, which only leaves the head, hands, and feet exposed, is made of tubes. During spacewalks, water flows through these tubes to keep the astronaut cool.

The Primary Life Support Subsystem backpack is located on the back of the spacesuit. The oxygen that astronauts use during spacewalks is kept in this backpack. Additionally, it eliminates the carbon dioxide astronauts exhale. The backpack also provides electricity for the outfit. The Liquid Cooling and Ventilation Garment's cooling water is stored in a water tank, and a fan circulates oxygen through the spacesuit and life support systems.

13. Which sentence describes how spacesuits keep users cool while on a spacewalk?

    A. Paragraph 1
    B. Paragraph 2
    C. Paragraph 3
    D. Paragraph 4

Answer: Paragraph 3

14. What feature of an astronaut's suit aids in appropriate breathing?

    A. Upper Torso Assembly,

    B. Upper Torso Assembly,

    C. Garment for liquid cooling and ventilation

    D. First Line of Life Support

Answer: First Line of Life Support

15. Which of these phrases best serves as a summary of the passage?

    A. An astronaut's spacesuit is considerably more than just a pair of garments they put on during spacewalks.

    B. The Gemini programme saw the first spacewalks ever conducted by NASA.

    C. Astronauts don the orange Advanced Crew Escape Suit when the space shuttle lifts off and touches down.

    D. NASA is also considering the components that spacesuits for missions to Mars will require.

Answer: An astronaut's spacesuit is considerably more than just a pair of garments they put on during spacewalks.

Passage

Eric is older than Ross

Erin is older than Rosanna

Rosanna is younger than Eric

16. Which of the following arrangements, ordered from oldest to youngest, is a possibility given the information above?

A. Erin, Rosanna, Eric, Ross

B. Eric, Rosanna, Erin, Ross

C. Ross, Erin, Eric, Rosanna

D. Eric, Ross, Erin, Rosanna

Answer: Eric, Ross, Erin, Rosanna

17. Which three income brackets collectively pay a payroll tax rate that is more than 29%?

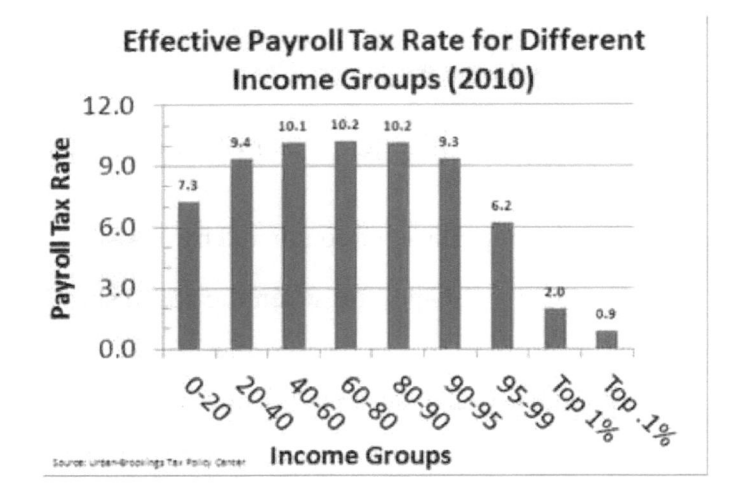

Effective Payroll Tax Rate for Different Income Groups (2010)

Income Group	Payroll Tax Rate
0–20	7.3
20–40	9.4
40–60	10.1
60–80	10.2
80–90	10.2
90–95	9.3
95–99	6.2
Top 1%	2.0
Top .1%	0.9

Source: Urban-Brookings Tax Policy Center

A. 0–20, 40–60, and 60–80

B. 20–40, 40–60, and 80–90

C. 20–40, 80–90, and 95–99

D. 40–60, 60–80, and Top 1%

Answer: 20–40, 40–60, and 80–90

Read and follow the directions below.

1. Start with a full deck of cards.
2. Remove all four jacks and four kings.

3. Add back in the red jacks.

4. Remove the eights.

5. Remove half the remaining cards at random.

18. Which of the following states how many cards are currently in the deck?

    A. 19

    B. 20

    C. 21

    D. 22

Answer: 21

Questions 19 to 20 are based on the following table.

Skin Type	At home in the UK	Europe and the Mediterranean	Florida/Africa/Caribbean
Very Fair/Sensitive	SPF 15 - 30	SPF 30 - 50	SPF 50+
Fair	SPF 15 - 20	SPF 30 - 50	SPF 50+
Normal	SPF 15	SPF 15 - 30	SPF 15 - 30
Olive	SPF 15	SPF 15	SPF 15 - 30
Dark	SPF 15	SPF 15	SPF 15 - 30
Children	SPF 30 - 50+	SPF 30 - 50+	SPF 30 - 50+

Source: Cancer Research UK

19. Trevor, who has exceptionally light complexion, intends to travel from his London home to Miami. How much should be added to the SPF of his sunscreen, at the very least?

    A. 20

B. 30

C. 40

D. 50

Answer:20

20. Based on the table, which statement is correct?

    A. In Europe, a fair-skinned person needs more than an SPF 30.

    B. A person with dark skin may need to use less sunscreen in the UK than in Africa.

    C. The Mediterranean is more sun-protective than the Caribbean for those with olive skin.

    D. When at home in the UK, children should use less sunscreen than fair-skinned persons.

Answer: A person with dark skin may need to use less sunscreen in the UK than in Africa.

Questions 21 to 22 are based on the following passage.

A blood glucose test, or fasting PG test, is given after a patient has gone without food for at least eight hours. It's widely considered to be a reliable test, and it appears the results aren't affected by patient age or physical activity. Many doctors prefer this method of testing because it's easy, fast and inexpensive.

21. In this context, reliable means

    A. noteworthy

    B. benign

    C. considerable

    D. accurate

Answer: accurate

22. Most often, a fasting PG test is used to:

    A. persuade people to consume less sugar;

    B. diagnose blood abnormalities that aren't picked up by other tests; or both.

    C. evaluate blood glucose levels.

    D. avoid paying for more expensive medical procedures

Answer: evaluate blood glucose levels.

Questions 23 to 27 are based on the following passage.

Thomas Paine is practically unknown compared to the majority of the other Founding Fathers of our nation. Many Americans, in fact, have never even heard of him. Paine was raised in a remote area of Thetford, England, as the son of a corsetier, a tailor who specialised in corsets and other undergarments. He was born in 1737. Young Paine held jobs as a corsetier, seaman, and clergyman before relocating to the British colonies in America, where he discovered his true calling.

As political unrest gripped the colonies, Paine initially rose to prominence as the editor of Pennsylvania Magazine. From there, he earned additional renown. Paine fervently campaigned for American independence from Britain in a book titled Common Sense that was published under an assumed name in 1776. The popularity of the book quickly reached 200,000 copies after taking off like wildfire. Paine released a collection of pamphlets titled The Crisis when the war started. These assisted in maintaining the soldiers' morale in the middle of a violent conflict. The phrase "The United States of America" is also given to Thomas Paine.

Thomas Jefferson and John Adams largely referenced Thomas Paine's writing when creating the Declaration of Independence because he was such a gifted writer. Later in life, Paine produced other, incredibly divisive writings. For his publications, he was even banished from England and imprisoned in France. Paine contributed to the creation of Social Security in 1796. In his final significant work, Agrarian Justice, he advocated for a system of social insurance for the young and the elderly.

23. Based on the passage's opening paragraph, which of the following conclusions makes sense?

    A. One of the Founding Fathers was Paine.

B. The American Revolution was ignited by the great writer Thomas Paine.

C. Without Paine's input, the Declaration of Independence could not have been written.

D. Paine's vast range of professional experiences certainly helped him form his political ideas.

Answer: One of the Founding Fathers was Paine.

24. What conclusion may be made about Thomas Paine's Common Sense based on the passage's second paragraph?

A. It was Thomas Paine's one and only meaningful contribution to the American Revolution.

B. It prompted King George to promise Thomas Paine retribution.

C. It was significantly influenced by his experience as a minister.

D. It was a driving force behind the American Revolution.

Answer: It was a driving force behind the American Revolution.

25. What is the passage's main argument by the author?

A. The American Revolution would not have occurred without Thomas Paine.

B. The contributions Thomas Paine contributed to the American Revolution should be honoured.

C. Even more significant than his earlier writings was Thomas Paine's later work.

D. Because Thomas Paine published his works anonymously, his achievements are not deserving of praise.

Answer: The contributions Thomas Paine contributed to the American Revolution should be honoured.

26. Which of the following passages may the reader deduce was the source of this one?

A. A political treatise

B. A history textbook

C. A tourist guidebook

D. A historical novel

Answer: A history textbook

27. Which of the following conclusions can be drawn by readers from the third paragraph's last sentences?

A. Thousands of people were motivated by Thomas Paine's Common Sense.

B. In his later years, Thomas Paine turned to crime.

C. The writings of Thomas Paine continue to have an impact on America.

D. Later in life, while incarcerated, Thomas Paine produced some of his greatest writings.

Answer: The writings of Thomas Paine continue to have an impact on America

Questions 28 to 29 are based on the following passage.

Wolfgang Amadeus Mozart had already produced five musical works by the age of five. Why are you holding out? The best day to start working toward something in your life is today, if you want to achieve it. Only those who are willing to take chances are rewarded by the universe. What's stopping you from becoming a legend, Mozart, who was only 5 years old?

28. Which of the following best bolsters the thesis in this section?

A. Stanford researchers claim that pursuing your passions will make you less successful in life.

B. Around the age of 30, Wolfgang Amadeus Mozart started to lose his hearing, and by the time he was 40, he was totally deaf.

C. At the age of seven, Pablo Picasso started receiving professional instruction in figure drawing and oil painting. His first words were "piz, piz," which is a shortened version of the Spanish term for pencil.

D. Early talent-showing children frequently fail to reach their full potential.

Answer: At the age of seven, Pablo Picasso started receiving professional instruction in figure drawing and oil painting. His first words were "piz, piz," which is a shortened version of the Spanish term for pencil.

29. Which of the following extra sentences, if this were an advertisement for a school or institution, would fit the best at the end of this passage?

A. You should start pursuing a career in medicine right away because the world needs more doctors.

B. No matter what you want out of life, education is necessary.

C. Mozart didn't wait, and neither should you.

D. Discover who you want to be by enrolling in our school right away.

Answer: Discover who you want to be by enrolling in our school right away.

Questions 30 to 32 are based on the following chart.

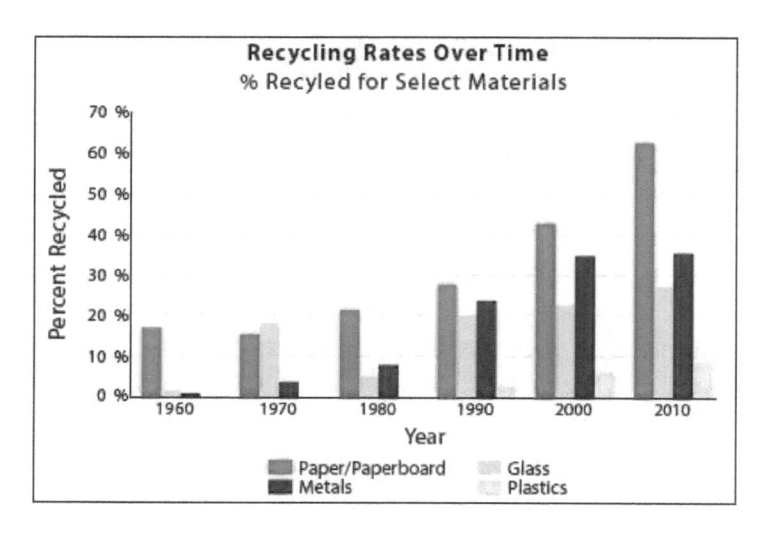

Recycling Rates Over Time
% Recyled for Select Materials

Paper/Paperboard Glass
Metals Plastics

30. What kind of substance has been recycled most frequently?

    A. paper

    B. metal

    C. glass

    D. cannot be determined from the chart

Answer: paper

31. What year did plastic recycling reach a level that was nearly 10%?

    A. 1980

    B. 1990

    C. 2000

    D. 2010

Answer: 2010

32. Which of the following inferences about the chart can be made with certainty?

    A. In contrast to earlier years, recycling of some products increased in 1960.

    B. The graph contains no information indicating whether recycling for any of the materials increased or decreased in 1960.

    C. Before 1960, recycling didn't exist.

    D. Recycling was not widely known in the years before 1960 among the general public.

Answer: The graph contains no information indicating whether recycling for any of the materials increased or decreased in 1960.

33. What is the patient's pulse rate based on the blood pressure cuff above?

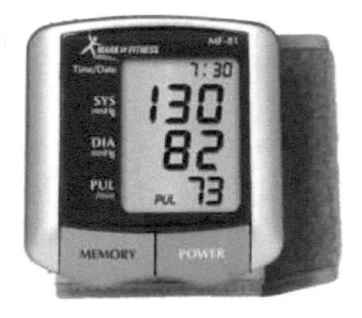

- A. 73
- B. 82
- C. 130/82
- D. 130

Answer: 73

34. Which type of intake should a client who consumes one of these prepared cookies likely limit for the rest of the day?

A. Saturated fat

B. Cholesterol

C. Carbohydrate

D. Fiber

Answer: Saturated fat

Passage

Some people's greatest accomplishments in adulthood must be attributed to the poverty and privations they experienced as children. At the age of thirteen, Robert Burns and his brother were expected to perform manly tasks. He had some formal education prior to then, and he must have advanced at that period because he had good reading and spelling skills in addition to some understanding of English grammar.

35. Which of the following would provide the best support for the claim made in the first line of the passage?

A. Despite receiving the best education money can buy, a young artist from a wealthy family does not find success as a painter.

B. A young author from a rural, underprivileged family wins a scholarship to a university, but she is unable to succeed.

C. C Despite coming from a working-class family, a child prodigy rises to fame as a violinist before reaching puberty.

D. A playwright is moved to create stunning plays about the poverty and challenges of his upbringing, and as a result, is widely recognised as the greatest writer of his generation.

Answer: A playwright is moved to create stunning plays about the poverty and challenges of his upbringing, and as a result, is widely recognised as the greatest writer of his generation.

36. What is the heaviest weight that this scale can detect?

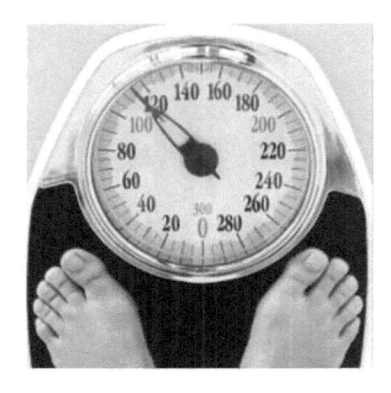

    A. 115 lbs.

    B. 28 lbs.

    C. 280 lbs.

    D. 300 lbs

Answer: 300 lbs

Passage

    Since we re-joined UNESCO, one of our primary goals has been to raise the literacy rate of our population, with a particular emphasis on the education of girls and women. To achieve this objective, effective informal education providers have played and will continue to play a vital role in the global effort to reduce the percentage of adults who are illiterate. We are aware that informal education can be more adaptive and help in reaching adults who have long since left the formal educational system or who were frequently denied access to it. This is something that can be accomplished with the help of technology. As the largest government donor to UNICEF, the United States is contributing to and supporting initiatives that aim to make schools safer and improve educational opportunities for all children, girls and boys alike.

37. Which of the following does the author of the aforementioned remarks not likely agree with

    A. Education of girls and women is sensible

    B. Education gives women more authority

    C. The value of formal education exceeds that of informal education

D. Girls and women should receive education

Answer: The value of formal education exceeds that of informal education

Questions 38 to 42 are based on the following passages.

Jonathan Swift's book Gulliver's Travels reflects his pessimistic view of humanity (1726). Swift was of the opinion that although society is supposed to shield individuals from inequity and injustice, it instead fosters the greatest vices, encourages immorality, and permits injustices to take place. Swift questions whether "civilization" is really a fancy name for the baser aspects of human nature in Gulliver's Travels.

Swift uses satire, a literary genre he perfects in Gulliver's Travels, to raise this question.

Following in the great tradition of classical satirists, Swift makes fun of society in his novel to highlight how absurd it really is. For instance, Gulliver portrays his own England to the monarch of a realm of giants in one chapter of Gulliver's Travels. Gulliver passionately discusses his country's social structure, laws, constitution, military might, and history with the enormous ruler. But after paying close attention to Gulliver's remarks, the monarch goes on to outline all of the problems with Gulliver's own country. Gulliver struggles to respond to the criticism in a suitable manner. As the king eventually decides that the institutions of the human world should be condemned, he can only watch in humiliated silence.

38. In the opening paragraph, the author conveys this idea by placing quote marks around the word "civilization."?

    A. skepticism

    B. wit

    C. anger

    D. studiousness

Answer: skepticism

39. In the text, the writer's argument mostly centres on

    A. The flaws of a civilisation

B. Swift's contempt for humanity

C. Swift's contempt for humanity

D. the source of Gulliver's character's inspiration

Answer: Swift's contempt for humanity

40. The passage implies that the giant king's opinion of England's laws and society is

    A. one of hidden jealously.

    B. close to Swift's own opinion.

    C. similar to the citizens of England's.

    D. in line with the author's own opinion.

Answer: close to Swift's own opinion.

41. Which of the following statements best describes the passage's point of view?

    A. In Gulliver's Travels, Gulliver talks with the ruler of the land of giants about politics and culture.

    B. A bleak view of humanity is presented in Gulliver's Travels.

    C. The most ideal example of Swift's satire is Gulliver's Travels.

    D. Gulliver is unable to respond to the king's criticisms in the land of giants in Gulliver's Travels.

Answer: The most ideal example of Swift's satire is Gulliver's Travels

42. The author would most likely agree that Swift

    A. was not involved with the English government

    B. uses satire to poke fun at human folly

    C. deliberately distorted historical facts for his own ends

D. believed that any attempt at human civilization should be abandoned

Answer: uses satire to poke fun at human folly

43. The scientific method is something that scientists must adhere to when conducting experiments. A framework for experimentation, the scientific method ensures reliable data. The goal of the experiment is the first step in the scientific method. What issue or question are they trying to answer? In order to ensure sure the experiment is worth the effort, they need then perform research to determine if anyone has already collected valid data on the subject. The data and the experimenters' prior knowledge are then used to develop a hypothesis or prediction of what will happen. Experimenters only need to carry out the experiment, gather the necessary data, and draw conclusions once the parameters and expectations have been made clear. If experimenters don't use this approach, they run the risk of tampering with their data and coming to false conclusions.

Which of the following best sums up the author's perspective?

A. In our daily lives, even if we are unaware of it, we all apply the scientific method.

B. The scientific method is used too frequently by experimenters without considering alternative approaches.

C. An experiment is deemed unsuccessful if it is unable to support the experimenter's hypothesis.

D. The best way to ensure that the results of your experiments are accurate and valid is to follow the scientific method.

Answer: The best way to ensure that the results of your experiments are accurate and valid is to follow the scientific method.

Passage 44 to 45

Cities all across the world are essentially amalgamations of more discrete cultural settings, which causes people to have incredibly diverse experiences. Every city often has a wide variety of food options as well as different art organisations like museums and theatres. What, then, can make a city stand out among all these variations in dining, art, and nightlife? History. Each city has an obviously distinctive past that fosters rich traditions and a sense of community that transcends the diversity of restaurants and cultural institutions found in other cities.

44. In context, which word most closely defines mélange?

    A. frivolous

    B. tradition

    C. assortment

    D. opportunity

Answer: assortment

45. Which of the following does the author consider to be the most significant city feature or attraction?

    A. The upscale French eatery in the European neighborhood

    B. The Natural History Museum

    C. Berlin Wall ruins as well as neighborhood ruins

    D. Wrigley Stadium

Answer: Berlin Wall ruins as well as neighborhood ruins

CHAPTER 2: Mathematics

The Mathematics section of the ATI TEAS (Test of Essential Academic Skills) exam assesses your knowledge and skills in various mathematical concepts. It covers a wide range of topics, including numbers and operations, data interpretation, algebra, and measurement. Here's a detailed discussion on how to prepare for the math test, with a focus on numbers and operations and data interpretation:

How to prepare for the math test:

a. Understand the Test Format: Familiarize yourself with the structure and format of the Mathematics section. The TEAS math test typically consists of around 36 questions, and you'll have 54 minutes to complete it. The questions are multiple-choice, and some might require you to perform calculations or solve problems.

b. Identify Weak Areas: Take a diagnostic practice test to identify your strengths and weaknesses in math. This will help you tailor your study plan to focus more on the topics you find challenging.

c. Review Math Concepts: Refresh your knowledge of fundamental math concepts, including arithmetic, algebra, geometry, and data interpretation. Make sure you have a good understanding of formulas and problem-solving techniques.

d. Practice Regularly: Consistent practice is essential to build confidence and improve your speed and accuracy. Work on a variety of practice questions and sample tests to simulate the exam environment.

e. Use Study Resources: Utilize study guides, textbooks, online tutorials, and other reliable resources to reinforce your understanding of math concepts. There are also specific TEAS preparation books available that focus on the exam's content.

f. Join Study Groups or Online Forums: Interacting with others preparing for the TEAS can be beneficial. Joining study groups or online forums can help you clarify doubts, share study tips, and learn from others' experiences.

g. Take Timed Practice Tests: Time management is crucial during the actual exam. Take timed practice tests to get used to the time pressure and develop strategies to pace yourself effectively.

h. Review Mistakes: After each practice test, carefully review the questions you answered incorrectly. Understand your errors, learn from them, and reinforce your weak areas.

Numbers and operations:

The Numbers and Operations category tests your understanding of basic arithmetic, fractions, decimals, percentages, ratios, and proportions. Here are some key topics to focus on:

a. Arithmetic Operations: Practice addition, subtraction, multiplication, and division of whole numbers, fractions, and decimals.

b. Fractions, Decimals, and Percentages: Learn to convert between fractions, decimals, and percentages. Practice operations involving fractions and decimals.

c. Ratios and Proportions: Understand the concept of ratios and proportions and how to solve problems using these concepts.

d. Order of Operations: Familiarize yourself with the order of operations (PEMDAS/BODMAS) to correctly solve complex mathematical expressions.

e. Estimation: Develop the skill of estimating results for numerical computations.

Data interpretation:

The Data Interpretation section assesses your ability to interpret data presented in various forms, such as charts, graphs, tables, and statistics. Here's how you can prepare for this section:

a. Chart and Graph Analysis: Practice interpreting information from bar graphs, line graphs, pie charts, scatter plots, and other types of graphs.

b. Table Analysis: Learn to extract relevant data from tables and use it to answer questions.

c. Statistics: Understand basic statistical concepts, such as mean, median, mode, range, and standard deviation, and apply them to interpret data.

d. Probability: Review probability concepts, such as calculating probabilities of events and understanding probability distributions.

e. Unit Conversion: Be proficient in converting units (e.g., length, weight, volume) and applying them to interpret data correctly.

Test Format:

The Mathematics section of the ATI TEAS exam assesses your mathematical knowledge and problem-solving abilities. It consists of around 36 multiple-choice questions and is timed for 54 minutes. The questions are designed to cover a wide range of mathematical concepts, including basic arithmetic, algebra, geometry, data interpretation, and measurement.

Content Areas:

The Mathematics section can be broadly categorized into several content areas:

a. Numbers and Operations: This area tests your understanding of fundamental arithmetic, fractions, decimals, percentages, ratios, and proportions.

b. Algebra: You may encounter questions related to solving equations, inequalities, and word problems that involve algebraic expressions and equations.

c. Geometry: This area covers concepts related to shapes, angles, area, perimeter, volume, and geometric principles.

d. Data Interpretation: You'll be required to analyze and interpret data presented in various forms, such as charts, graphs, tables, and statistics.

e. Measurement: Questions in this area involve converting units, working with measurements, and solving problems related to time, distance, speed, and other quantitative measures.

How to Prepare for the Mathematics Section:

To excel in the Mathematics section of the ATI TEAS exam, follow these preparation tips:

a. Review Fundamentals: Start by revisiting core math concepts, including basic arithmetic, fractions, decimals, percentages, and algebraic operations. Make sure you have a strong foundation before moving on to more advanced topics.

b. Practice Regularly: Consistent practice is key to building confidence and improving your problem-solving skills. Work on a variety of practice questions and sample tests to become familiar with the exam format and types of questions you might encounter.

c. Utilize Study Materials: Utilize study guides, textbooks, online tutorials, and TEAS-specific preparation resources. There are dedicated TEAS prep books and online courses available that focus on the content and format of the exam.

d. Take Timed Practice Tests: Simulate the exam environment by taking timed practice tests. This will help you develop time-management strategies and get used to the time pressure during the actual exam.

e. Identify Weak Areas: After taking practice tests, identify your areas of weakness and focus on improving them. Concentrate more on topics where you face challenges and need more practice.

f. Understand Data Interpretation: The data interpretation questions often challenge test-takers. Practice analyzing charts, graphs, and tables to improve your ability to extract relevant information and answer questions accurately.

g. Memorize Formulas: While the TEAS may provide some basic formulas, it's a good idea to memorize common mathematical formulas to save time during the exam.

h. Stay Calm and Confident: On the day of the exam, stay calm and confident. Trust in your preparation and don't let difficult questions fluster you. If you encounter a challenging question, consider marking it for review and move on to the next one. You can always come back to it later.

4. Importance of the Mathematics Section: The Mathematics section in the ATI TEAS exam is essential because it evaluates your mathematical proficiency, which is crucial for success in various healthcare-related fields. As a prospective nursing or allied health program student, you'll need to handle medication dosages, perform basic calculations, and interpret numerical data regularly. Strong math skills are essential to ensure patient safety and accurate healthcare procedures.

The ATI TEAS exam assesses your understanding of various mathematical concepts, including Measurement and Data, Geometry, and general Mathematics questions. Let's discuss each of these topics in detail, along with the importance of detailed answer keys for your preparation.

Measurement and data:

The Measurement and Data category in the ATI TEAS exam evaluates your ability to work with measurements and interpret data. This section includes questions related to converting units, calculating measurements, and solving problems involving time, distance, speed, and other quantitative measures. It also involves analyzing and interpreting data presented in the form of charts, graphs, tables, and statistics.

a. Measurement Concepts: Review the conversion between different units, such as length, weight, volume, and temperature. Practice solving measurement-related problems involving units.

b. Time and Distance: Practice questions that require you to calculate time, speed, and distance, especially in the context of real-life scenarios.

c. Data Interpretation: Work on questions that involve analyzing and interpreting information presented in various forms, such as bar graphs, line graphs, pie charts, and tables.

d. Statistics: Understand basic statistical concepts, including mean, median, mode, range, and standard deviation. Be prepared to apply these concepts to interpret data.

Geometry:

The Geometry section tests your knowledge of shapes, angles, area, perimeter, volume, and geometric principles. Some key topics to focus on include:

a. Geometric Shapes: Review properties and characteristics of common geometric shapes, such as triangles, circles, squares, rectangles, and polygons.

b. Angles: Understand different types of angles, such as acute, obtuse, right, and straight angles. Practice angle calculations and relationships between angles.

c. Area and Perimeter: Learn how to calculate the area and perimeter of various shapes, including squares, rectangles, triangles, and circles.

d. Volume: Be familiar with formulas to calculate the volume of 3D shapes like cubes, cylinders, and spheres.

e. Geometric Principles: Understand concepts like congruence, similarity, and symmetry.

Questions & Answers

1. Which one of the following percentages is the same as 0.0016?

a) 0.0016%

b) 16%

c) 1.6%

d) 0.16%

Answer: D. 0.16%.

In this case the sum is 0.0016 x 100 = 0.16%

2. Emilia is driving through Russia which uses metric measurements for distance signs.

a) 31 miles

b) 37 miles

c) 48 miles

d) 22 miles

Answer: A. 31 miles.

One kilometer is equivalent to around 0.62 miles. Multiply 50 km by 0.62 miles to give you 31 miles.

3. Simon scored the following grades on his last seven mathematics exams: 93, 80, 91, 88, 85 82 and 92. What is his approximate average score?

a) 89

b) 81

c) 87

d) 92

Answer: C. 87.

To find the average score of Simon's grades you must add all the six grades (93 + 80 +91 + 88 + 85 + 82 + 92) and divide the total by six (the number of scores). 93 + 80 +91 + 88 + 85 + 82 + 92 = 611. 611 divided by 7 is equal to 87.2. The approximation of 87.2 to the nearest whole number is 87.

4. What is the median of Simon's scores?

a) 88

b) 90

c) 91

d) 82

Answer: A. 88.

The median is found by arranging the scores from the lowest to the highest score and finding the number in the middle. In this case the scores from the lowest to the highest are: 80, 82, 85, 88, 91, 92, 93. So, the median number is the middle number which is 88.

5. Ian wants to shop for jackets since winter is just around the corner. He has identified two jackets at the local men's clothing store. The store advertises that the jackets, among other clothing, are on sale and there is an incentive: 25% off every second item of less or equal value. One Jacket costs $60 and the second one is $50. Ian purchases both jackets. How much does he spend?

a) $97.50

b) $83

c) $110

d) $87.50

Answer: A. $97.50.

The sale discount will be applied on the jacket that costs less which is the $50 jacket. 25% off $50 is $12.50. That means that Ian will only pay $37.50 for this jacket. But the first jacket doesn't get discounted so it remains $60. Ian's total spend will be $60 + $37.50 = $97.50.

6. You need to buy pens and printing paper for your students. If one pen costs $30 and one ream of paper is $5, which of the following answer choices offers the correct sum of your purchases out of $100.

a) 30c + 5p ≥ 100

b) 30c + 5p ≤ 100

c) 30c + 5p > 100

d) 30c + 5p < 100

Answer: B. 30c + 5p ≤ 100.

The amount you spend will be less than or equal to $100 because if you go over $100, you will be short of money to pay for the pens and paper.

7. Pierre wanted to purchase a computer from the local electronics shop. The unit he chose was on sale with a 30% discount on its original price which was $472. What is the final price that Pierre paid for the computer?

a) $141.60

b) $330.40

c) $472

d) $500

Answer: B. 30/100 X 472 = 141.60. So, the discount is $141.60. When you subtract $141.60 from $472 you get $330.40. Pierre paid $330.40 for the computer after the discount.

8. On a construction site, the foreman needs to load four wheelbarrows of construction into an elevator that has a 900-pound weight limit. What would the average weight of each of the wheelbarrows be if the foreman is 200 pounds, and he must accompany the equipment without going over the elevator's weight limit.

a) 150 pounds

b) 128 pounds

c) 180 pounds

d) 175 pounds

Answer: D. 175 pounds.

Begin by subtracting the foreman's weight from the 900-pound limit, 900 − 200 = 700. You have to fit the remaining weight within the remaining 700-pound limit. Divide the 600 pounds by the four wheelbarrows, 700 ÷ 4 = 175 pounds. Each wheelbarrow will carry an average weight of 175 pounds.

9. Omar is going on a self-funded business trip. He has added up the cost of the trip according to the following breakdown. The airfare will be $675, roundtrip. His hotel room per night is $89 per night and he intends to be in town for five nights. He has allocated $200 for transportation around the city to meetings and $250 for meals. At the hotel, he is offered a discount of 10% off the $89 per night for subsequent nights after the first night. How much is Omar going to spend on this trip?

a) $1534.40

b) $409.40

c) $1125

d) $675

Answer: A. $1534.40.

Begin by adding up the other costs of the trip excluding the room. That is 675 + 200 + 250 = $1125. Next calculate how much Omar will pay for his accommodation. The five nights are supposed to cost her $89 per night but since she is receiving a 10% discount on the four nights after her first night, she will pay $89 for the first night and 80.1 per night for the remaining four nights. Therefore, her accommodation will be 89 + 80.1 + 80.1 + 80.1 + 80.1 = $409.40. Now add the total for the room cost to the total of the other costs of the trip for the overall total Omar will spend. 1125 + 409.40 = $1534.40 Omar will spend $1534.40 on his trip.

10. While skiing on the ski slope Emma tumbled 20 out of the 27 times she tried to ski. What percentage of times did Emma tumble and fall?

a) 74% of the time

b) 26% of the time

c) 50% of the time

d) 90% of the time

Answer: A. 74% of the time.

Emma fell 20 out of 27 times. So to find the answer in percentage divide 20 by 27 and then multiply the answer by 100. 20 ÷ 27 = 0.740 X 100 = 74%.

11. Charity received a gift measuring a length of 14 inches with a height of 8 inches and 6 inches in width.

a) 244

b) 680

c) 488

d) 67

Answer: C. 488.

Using the formula SA = 2lw + 2wh + 2hl, you will substitute the letters for the dimensions of the box like this: SA = 2 (14) (6) + 2 (6) (8) + 2 (8) (14) = 488 square inches.

12. Michael received a bonus at work at the end of the year. From the bonus he gave 30% to a charity organization, paid 30% in taxes, and paid a debt with 25%. He was left with $450 from the initial bonus money. How much was Michael's bonus?

a) $3600

b) $3200

c) $3000

d) $4000

Answer: D. $3000.

In total Michael paid out 85% of his bonus (30% + 30% + 25%). That leaves him with only 15%. If 15% is 600 then 100/15 X 600 will give you the answer that is $3000.

13. Mariah's current weight is 65 kilograms. If one kilogram is equivalent to 2.2 pound, approximate her weight in pounds.

a) Mariah is exactly 143 pounds

b) Mariah is approximately 123 pounds

c) Mariah is approximately 160 pounds

d) Mariah is approximately 187 pounds

Answer: A. Mariah is exactly 143 pounds.

The answer is 65 kilograms multiplied by 2.2 pounds which is 143 pounds. That is Stella's weight.

14. One of the following integers is listed from the least to the greatest. Which one is the correct combination?

a) -3/4, -7 4/5, -8, 18%, 0.25, 2.5

b) -8, -7 4/5, -3/4, 0.25, 2.5. 18%

c) 18%, 0.25, -3/4, 2.5, -7 4/5, -8

d) -8, -7 4/5, -3/4, 18%, 0.25, 2.5

Answer: D. -8, -7 4/5 -3/4, 18%, 0.25, 2.5.

Remember the integers with the smallest negative value tend to have the largest absolute value. As such, the negative integers -7 4/5, -8, -3/4 have the least value. 18% converted into a decimal value becomes 0.18 which is smaller than 0.25. 2.5 is the greatest rational number in the group.

15. According to census records, the number of births in the small town of Kiria increased from 1500 to 2400. Find the approximate percentage increase in the number of births during this period.

a) Add 1500 + 2400 = 3900, then divide the result 3900 by 1500 to get the percentage increase and then multiply by 100 to get the percentage. Finally, approximate the final figure.

b) Add 1500 + 2400 = 3900, then divide the result 3900 by 2400 to get the percentage increase and then multiply by 100 to get the percentage. Finally, approximate the final figure.

c) Subtract 1500 from 2400 = 900, then divide the result 900 by 1500 to get the percentage increase and then multiply by 100 to get the percentage. Finally, approximate the final figure.

d) Multiply 1500 + 2400 = 3900, then divide the result 3900 by 1500 to get the percentage increase and then multiply by 100 to get the percentage. Finally, approximate the final figure.

Answer: C. Subtract 1500 from 2400 = 900, then divide the result 900 by 1500 to get the percentage increase and then multiply by 100 to get the percentage. Finally, approximate the final figure.

2400 -1500 = 900. 900 ÷ 1500 = 0.6 x 100 = 60%. You will notice the number 60% is complete. But if there was a decimal number like 60.8, then the approximate number is 61%.

16. The following expression can be simplified. How? 2.401 x 0.0178 =

a) 2.0358414

b) 0.0427378

c) 0.2341695

d) 0.3483240

Answer: B. 0.0427378.

This is a multiplication problem so the answer should simply come from multiplying 2.401 x 0.0178 = 0.0427378

17. A rectangular room of 30 cm2 is converted into a drawn floor plan at a scale of 1:100.

a) 30,000 cm2

b) 3,000 m2

c) 300 m2

d) 30 m

Answer: D. 30 m.

There are 100 cm in every meter so on a 1:100 scale drawing each one centimeter represents a meter. That means the area of one sq cm (square centimeter) on the drawing should represent one square meter in actuality. And because the area of the room on the drawing scale is 30 cm2, the room's actual area is typically 30 m2.

18. Solve the following problems. Find x in 2x + 4 = x-6

a) X = - 12

b) X = 10

c) X = - 16

d) X = - 10

Answer: D. X = - 10.

To solve the equation, begin by subtracting the four on both sides of the sum. 2x + 4 -4 = x-6 – 4 leaving you with 2x = x – 10, then eliminate the x on both sides of the equation 2x -x = x – 10 – x and the answer is X = -10 Find x in 2x – 7 = 3 a) X = 4 b) X = -2 c) X = 5 d) X = 3 Answer: C. 5. To solve the equation begin by adding 7 on both sides of the sum. 2x – 7 + 7 = 3 + 7 leaving you with 2x = 10 then divide it by two 2x/2 = 10/2 resulting in X = 5

19. Simplify this expression: ¼ x 3/5 ÷ 1 1/8 = ?

a) 8/15

b) 2/15

c) 27/160

d) 27/40

Answer: B. 2/15.

This equation should be solved in order of operations. So, begin with the ¼ x 3/5 = 3/20 and then follow it up with the division section which requires you to reverse the fraction. Therefore, the division section should be 3/20 ÷ 9/8, alternatively it can be 3/20 x 8/9 which equals 24/180. Simplify this further to 2/15. So, the answer is 2/15.

20. Calculate the ratio of yellow to green cars in the car park if there are 120 yellow cars and 230 green cars.

a) 23: 35

b) 12: 23

c) 35: 12

d) 13: 23

Answer: A. 23: 35.

The first part of the ratio must indicate the 230 green cars and the second part should indicate the total sum of the green and yellow cars. The ratio should therefore look like this: 230:350 so that when it is simplified it results in 23:35.

21. If a five-centimeter line represents four kilometers on the road, what is the length of the road represented by eight centimeters?

a) 10 km

b) 64 km

c) 6.4 km

d) 2.0 km

Answer: C. 6.4 km.

If 5 cm represent 4 km that means that 1 cm is equivalent to 4/5 of a kilometer. So, 8 centimeters is multiplied by 4/5 of a kilometer to result in 6.4 km. The sum should look like this: 4/5 X 8/1 = 32/5 which when converted into decimals is 6.4.

22. A company making a total profit and loss a week needs you to calculate the overall profit or loss it actually makes. On Monday and Tuesday, they report a loss of $300, a loss of $100 on Wednesday, but make a profit of $400 on Thursdays and $600 profits on Friday and Saturday.

a) $1400

b) $600

c) $2300

d) $900

Answer: D. $900.

Create an expression with the figures you have been given. (-$300 + -$300 + -$100 + $600 + %600 + $400) and that will give you $900.

23. Calculate the following simple mathematical problem 4 + 6 - 11 + 2

a) 1

b) 7

c) 3

d) 11

Answer: A. 1.

24. Solve this equation: -6x = 36

a) -6

b) 216

c) 30

d) -30

Answer: A. - 6.

36 and 6 are both divisible by the common denominator which is 6. So divide both sides of the equation by six to arrive at x = - 6.

25. Solve the below equation. 3 (y +1) + 2(y+1) > 5 (3-y) + 4 (y + 2)

a) Y = -5

b) Y = 3

c) Y = 8

d) Y = -3

Answer: B. y = 3.

Begin by solving the equation on both sides of the greater than sign so that $3(y+1) + 2(y+1)$ becomes $3y + 2y + 2 = 5y + 5$. And the $5(3-y) + 4(y+2)$ is solved to become $15 - 5y + 4y + 8 = 23 - y$ Now the equation is $5y + 5 > 23 - y$. Get rid of the like terms on each side of this equation so that it becomes $6y + 5 > 23$. Go ahead to subtract 5 from the 23 because these are like terms so that you remain with $6y > 18$. Simplify the sum further by dividing the terms by a common denominator which in this case is 6. The result is $y = 3$.

CHAPTER 3: The Science

Body systems:

Your knowledge of the many body systems, which are sets of organs and tissues that work together to execute certain functions in the body, may be evaluated as part of the ATI TEAS Test. The following are examples of important body systems that may be covered on the test:

• The Respiratory System: This is the part of the body that is in charge of exchanging gases (oxygen and carbon dioxide) with the outside world. Lungs, trachea, and bronchi are some of the organs that are included in this system.

• The Circulatory System, sometimes referred to as the Cardiovascular System, is in charge of moving blood, nutrients, and oxygen across the body. It is also known as the cardiovascular system. It comprises the heart as well as the blood arteries and the blood itself.

• The digestive system is responsible for breaking down food, absorbing its nutrients, and getting rid of its waste products. The stomach, the small intestine, and the large intestine are all considered organs.

• The Muscular System: Responsible for the body's mobility and structural integrity. It encompasses the skeletal muscles, as well as the smooth and cardiac muscles.

• The skeletal system is responsible for providing organs with both structural support and protection. It is made up of skeletal tissue, cartilage, and joint cartilage.

• The Nervous System: This system regulates the functioning of the body and reacts to both internal and external stimuli. It encompasses the head as well as the spinal cord and the nerves.

• The endocrine system is responsible for regulating the functions of the body by secreting hormones. It is composed of glands such as the pituitary gland, the thyroid gland, and the adrenal glands.

• The reproductive system is the part of the body that is in charge of creating offspring. In males, it is comprised of the testes and the penis, whereas in females, it is comprised of the ovaries and the uterus.

- The Integumentary System: This system helps maintain a normal body temperature while also protecting the body from potential dangers from the outside world. It encompasses the hair, nails, and skin as well.

Transportation based on individual cells:

The movement of substances (molecules, ions, and so on) through the membranes of individual cells is referred to as cell-based transportation. This process is necessary for the continuation of cellular life as well as the proper functioning of the organism as a whole. There are primarily two different kinds of transportation that are based on cells:

- Passive Transport: This method of transport does not need any additional expenditure of energy on the part of the cell. This includes the following:

- Diffusion is the process by which molecules move from a region of high concentration to a region of low concentration until equilibrium is achieved.

- Osmosis is the process in which water molecules migrate over a semi-permeable membrane from a region where there is a lower concentration of solutes to a region where there is a higher concentration of solutes.

- Active Transport: In order to move substances against their concentration gradient (from low to high concentration), this type of transport necessitates the use of energy, which often takes the form of ATP. The sodium-potassium pump and endocytosis/exocytosis are two examples of such processes.

cellular nucleus

The word "nuclear cell" appears to have multiple meanings, and the notion itself is not well defined in the field of biology. It's likely that this phrase is referring to a cell that has a nucleus, in which case it would apply to practically all eukaryotic cells (cells that have a clearly defined nucleus that's surrounded by a membrane). There are eukaryotic cells in all multicellular organisms, including plants, mammals, fungi, and protists.

Eukaryotic cells are distinguished from prokaryotic cells, which include bacteria and archaea, by the existence of a nucleus, which is a defining trait of eukaryotic cells. On the other hand, prokaryotic cells do not include a genuine nucleus. Instead, it is located in a part of their cell called the nucleoid, which is responsible for storing their DNA.

Anatomy and physiology of the human body

The disciplines of human anatomy and physiology are academic fields that investigate the relationship between the structure and function of the human body. It entails having a grasp of how the different bodily systems interact with one another to keep homeostasis and sustain life. The following is a list of important subjects that might be discussed in this area:

• Tissues is the study of several types of tissues, including epithelial, connective, muscular, and neurological tissues, among others.

• Organs: An understanding of the structure and function of key organs, including the heart, lungs, liver, and brain, amongst others.

• Systems: Extensive understanding of the body's various systems, including their underlying anatomical structures and the physiological processes that they support.

• Homeostasis is the capacity of the organism to keep the internal environment stable in spite of changes in the external environment.

Cycle of the heart

The term "cardiac cycle" refers to the series of events that take place throughout the entirety of a single heartbeat. In order to move blood through the circulatory system, the chambers of the heart, known as the atria and ventricles, contract and relax in a cycle known as the cardiac cycle. The following are the primary stages of the cardiac cycle:

• Atrial Contraction (Atrial Systole): During this phase of the heart's rhythm, the atria squeeze together, which forces blood into the ventricles.

• Ventricular Contraction (Ventricular Systole): During this phase of the heart's beating, the ventricles contract, which forces blood to be pumped out of the heart. While the left ventricle is responsible for pumping blood to the rest of the body (systemic circulation), the right ventricle is responsible for pumping blood to the lungs (pulmonary circulation).

• During the period of relaxation known as diastole, the muscles of the heart become more relaxed, and blood from the veins begins to fill the atria.

An electrocardiogram (also known as an ECG or EKG) can be used to monitor and record electrical impulses that are produced by the heart's conduction system. These impulses are responsible for regulating the cardiac cycle.

Electrocardiogram

An electrocardiogram, often known as an ECG or EKG, is a diagnostic procedure that records the electrical activity of the heart over the course of an extended period of time. It is an important diagnostic technique that is used to evaluate the health of the heart and find anomalies in the rhythm of the heart. The electrical impulses that are produced by the heart's conduction system as it contracts and relaxes are what are measured by the electrocardiogram (ECG).

The electrocardiogram is displayed in the form of a graph that contains characteristic waveforms, each of which represents a different phase of the heart cycle. The P-wave, also known as atrial depolarization, the QRS complex, also known as ventricular depolarization, and the T-wave, sometimes known as ventricular repolarization, are the primary components of an electrocardiogram waveform.

Abnormalities in the electrocardiogram can be indicators of a variety of cardiac disorders, including arrhythmias, myocardial infarction (also known as a heart attack), and hypertrophy of either the atrium or ventricles.

Neurological apparatus

The nervous system is made up of a vast network of specialized cells known as neurons, which are responsible for relaying chemical and electrical impulses throughout the body. It is possible to roughly separate it into two primary components:

• The brain and spinal cord are both components of the Central Nervous System (CNS). The processing of information and the coordination of replies are both under its purview.

• The Peripheral Nervous System, often known as the PNS, is made up of nerves that branch out from the Central Nervous System and connect to the remainder of the body. The PNS can be further subdivided into the somatic nervous system and the autonomic nervous system. The somatic nervous system is in charge of voluntary movement, while the autonomic nervous system regulates involuntary functions such as heart rate and digestion.

The nervous system is extremely important for the processes of maintaining homeostasis, as well as sensory perception and motor control. It enables us to react to stimuli from the outside world, process information, and engage in conversation with our surroundings.

Question & Answers

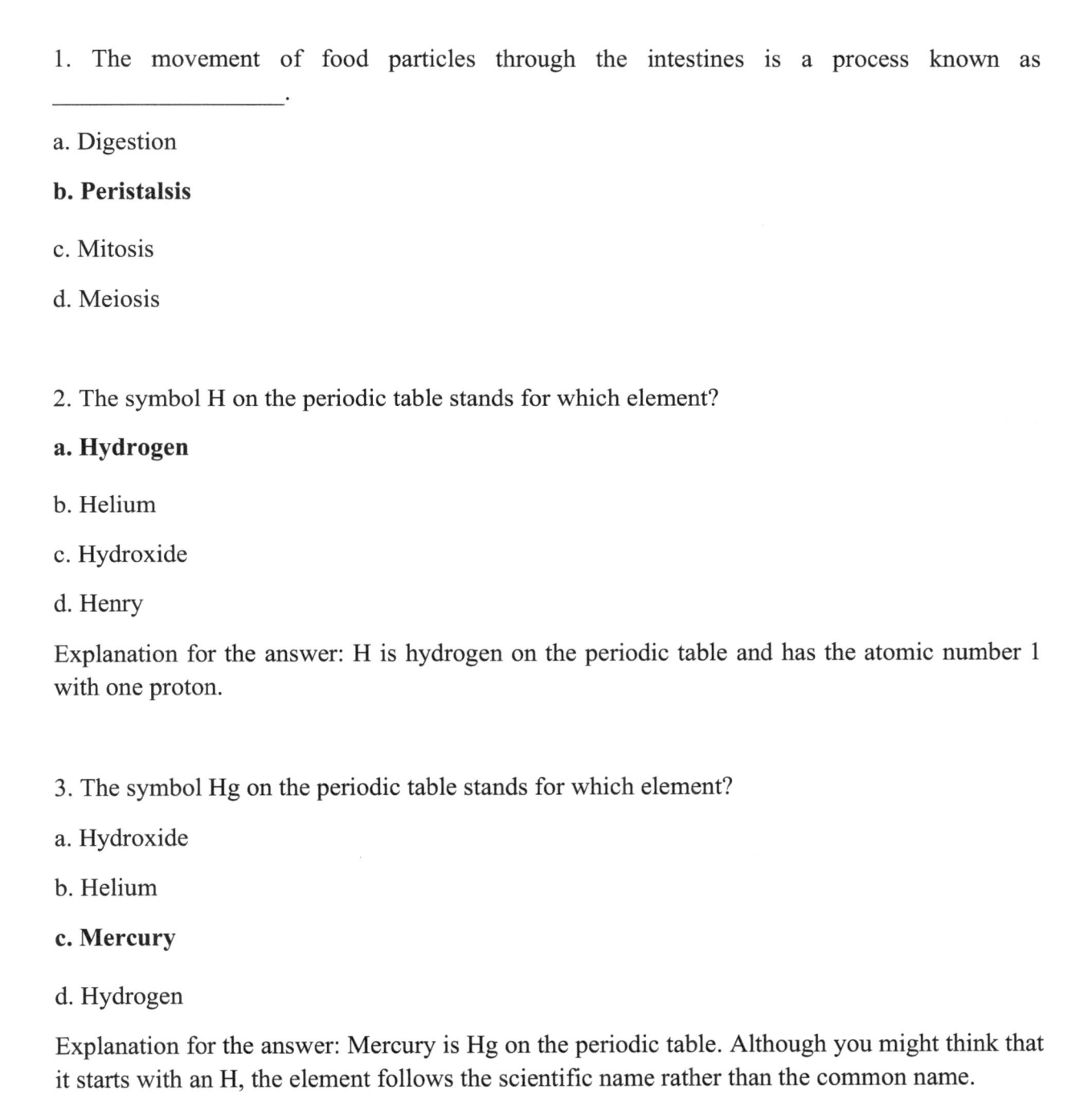

1. The movement of food particles through the intestines is a process known as _____.

a. Digestion

b. Peristalsis

c. Mitosis

d. Meiosis

2. The symbol H on the periodic table stands for which element?

a. Hydrogen

b. Helium

c. Hydroxide

d. Henry

Explanation for the answer: H is hydrogen on the periodic table and has the atomic number 1 with one proton.

3. The symbol Hg on the periodic table stands for which element?

a. Hydroxide

b. Helium

c. Mercury

d. Hydrogen

Explanation for the answer: Mercury is Hg on the periodic table. Although you might think that it starts with an H, the element follows the scientific name rather than the common name.

4. This is a type of reaction that releases heat and light energy.

a. Exothermic

b. Endothermic

c. Helium

d. Explosion

Explanation for the answer: An exothermic reaction releases heat and energy. In this reaction, the heat is all used up by the reaction.

5. The combination of sodium and chlorine to form sodium chloride (NaCl), which is table salt, is called a/an _____ bond.

a. Ionic

b. Covalent

c. Helium

d. Explosion

Explanation for the answer: With ionic compounds, you have one proton and electron, which are exchanged, and that is what happens in this reaction. Na has +1 charge and Cl has −1 charge. And with opposites, they attract and form this compound.

6. _____ electrons are responsible for chemical reactions and the creation of compounds.

a. Vector

b. Hybrid

c. Valence

d. Special

Explanation for the answer: Valence electrons are ones that occur on the outer shell of an atom. And they are responsible for the chemical reactions.

7. _____ is a phase in which chromosomes form a line during mitosis.

a. Telophase

b. Anaphase

c. Prophase

d. Metaphase

8. Which of the following statements is true about enzymes?

a. Enzymes are destroyed during chemical reactions.

b. Enzymes are all harmful.

c. Almost all enzymes are proteins.

d. Enzymes are not helpful to humans.

9. Lipids are composed of _____.

a. Zinc

b. Nutrients

c. Fatty acids

d. White blood cells

10. Down syndrome affects which of the following chromosomes?

a. 20

b. 21

c. 23

d. 25

11. The abuse of alcohol is linked with the cancer of which organ?

a. Liver

b. Stomach

c. Kidney

d. Heart

Explanation for the answer: The liver is an organ that is deeply affected by the use and abuse of alcohol. It has been linked with liver failure as well as cancer.

12. Animals that are known for eating exclusively plants are called _____.

a. Carnivores

b. Omnivores

c. Herbivores

d. Mammals

Explanation for the answer: Herbivores are plant-eating organisms. Omnivores eat both plants and meat, whereas carnivores eat only meat. Finally, mammals are a class of animals.

13. A car is driving at a constant velocity of 50 m/s and has been traveling for more than 2 min. What is the acceleration of the car?

a. 0

b. 23 m/s

c. 25 m/s

d. 40 m/s2

14. Neurons are joined together at points known as _____.

a. Terminals

b. Junction

c. Joint

d. Synapse

15. The organ known as the corti is found in which area of the body?

a. Lungs

b. Heart

c. Ear

d. Mouth

16. Which of the following functions is not performed by the kidneys?

a. Reabsorption

b. Filtration

c. Transportation

d. Secretion

17. In the colors of the rainbow, ROYGBIV, which color is V?

a. Verdure

b. Village

c. Velocity

d. Violet

18. The scientific name for vinegar is _____.

a. Acetic acid

58 | ATI TEAS

b. Sulfuric acid

c. Acetone acid

d. Ascorbic acid

19. How would you write the scientific name for water?

a. hydroxide

b. hydrogen dioxide

c. hydrogen sulfide

d. Nitrogen dioxide

20. These are forces that can be shown on graph paper by using _____.

a. Slopes

b. Triangles

c. Vectors

d. Variables

21. What is the name of the gaps between neurons?

a. Cell voids

b. Synapses

c. Inter-neurons

d. Dendrites

22. During pulmonary circulation, which of the following heart chambers receives blood coming back from the lungs?

a. Right atrium

b. Left ventricle

c. **Left atrium**

d. Right ventricle

23. Which of the following statements accurately sums up a strong acid?

a. At least one metal atom can be found in a strong acid.

b. Strong acids cannot break down.

c. More than one proton is donated by a potent acid.

d. **In water, a strong acid totally ionises.**

24. Which of the following will be brought on by an aortic dissection?

a. The heart would not get deoxygenated blood.

b. The lungs wouldn't receive deoxygenated blood.

c. The atria of the heart would not receive oxygenated blood.

d. **The body's cells could not receive oxygenated blood.**

25. Which of the following describes the respiratory system's inhaling process the best?

a. The air pressure in the lungs decreases as a result of the diaphragm lifting and contracting.

b. The air pressure in the lungs rises as the diaphragm loosens and raises.

c. **The air pressure in the lungs decreases as a result of the diaphragm's contraction and descent.**

d. The air pressure in the lungs decreases as the diaphragm loosens and drops.

26. Which of the following is the anterior bone of the lower leg?

a. **Tibia**

b. Fibula

c. Radius

d. Ulna

27. What environment produces immune cells?

a. Liver

b. **Bone marrow**

c. Thymus

d. Lymph nodes

28. Which of the following describes the cartilaginous flap that shields the larynx from food and liquids while maintaining airflow?

a. Bronchioles

b. **Epiglottis**

c. Tongue

d. Epithelium

29. Which of the following best describes the movement of an action potential along a neuron's axon?

a. Electrical transmission

b. Chemical reactivity

c. Repolarization

d. **Saline conductivity**

30. Which of the following reactions results in decomposition?

a. Zn + 2hcl → zncl2 + H2

b. 2Na + Cl2 → 2nacl

c. H2CO3 → H2O + CO2

d. CH4 + 2O2 → CO2 +2H2O

31. What kind of bond binds oxygen and hydrogen atoms together to form water molecules?

a. Covalent bond

b. Ionic bond

c. Metallic bond

d. Hydrogen bond

32. Which of the following describes the bonds that bind nonpolar covalent molecules together?

a. They can only be created between two atoms that are the same.

b. They can only be created between two distinct atoms.

c. They occur when two atoms share a pair of electrons with each other

d. They take place when two atoms share a pair of metal ions.

33. Which of the following atmospheric layers is nearest to outer space?

a. Troposphere

b. Stratosphere

c. Mesosphere

d. Thermosphere

34. Which of the following best sums up how cytokines generally work within the immune system?

a. They prevent blood clotting when the body is responding to inflammation.

b. To enhance pathogen bulk, they bind to particular infections.

c. They interact with one another in order to trigger an immunological response.

d. They move germs that are mucus-trapped and will be eliminated in the stomach.

35. Which statement about anatomical position is accurate?

a. Standing straight with arms at sides and palms front

b. Sitting with arms at sides and palms facing backward

c. Supine with arms at sides and hands facing backward

d. Supine with arms at sides and hands facing forward

36. Which of the following best describes the order in which an inflammatory reaction takes place?

I. Phagocytes are drawn to the area that is injured.

II. Blood vessels start to leak.

III. Histamine is released by damaged cells.

IV. Pus starts to develop

a. IV, I, III, II

b. I, III, II, IV

c. III, II, I, IV

d. II, I, III, IV

37. Which of the following is thought to have played a role in the decline in newborn mortality in developed nations?

a. The mother's marital status.

b. The chances for women to pursue education.

c. The rise in medical expenses

d. The decrease in domestic abuse directed at expectant mothers.

38. By storing adipocytes and releasing them into circulation when energy is required, which of the following skin layers serves as an energy reserve?

a. Dermis

b. Hypodermis

c. Epidermis

d. Stratum basale

39. Which of the following structures does air pass through after entering the mouth, nose, and throat?

a. Trachea

b. Bronchioles

c. Bronchi

d. Alveoli

40. Which cell in the list below contains oxygen?

a. Thrombocytes

b. Leukocytes

c. **Erythrocytes**

d. Plasma cells

41. Which of the following chemical bond types is present in hexane?

a. Bonding in two and threes

b. **Single bonds only**

c. Triple and single bonds

d. Solitary and double bonds

42. After Order, whose taxonomic level is the smallest?

a. Genus

b. **Family**

c. Species

d. Phylum

43. Which of the following would be less limiting than an organism's family under Linnaeus' classification scheme?

a. Genus

b. Taxon

c. Species

d. **Order**

44. How many additional electrons are required for the halogens' valence shell to be complete?

a. 7

b. **1**

c. 6

d. 2

45. Which of the following would be the most appropriate unit of measurement for an experiment to determine the amount that people of different ages can exhale?

a. Atm

b. **Liters**

c. Amu

d. Grams

46. Two separate beakers are used to conduct the identical single-replacement reaction. Beaker A and Beaker B are the designated beakers, and they are heated to 75°C and 100°C, respectively. Which of the following outcomes would you anticipate to see if the reactions are run for each one for 15 minutes?

a. **More product is produced by Beaker B than by Beaker A.**

b. In either beaker, no products are created.

c. More product is produced by Beaker A than by Beaker B.

d. The amount of product produced by the two beakers is equal.

47. Which of the following elements has an atomic radius that is the largest?

a. Strontium (Sr)

b. Calcium (Ca)

c. **Barium (Ba)**

d. Magnesium (Mg)

48. The experiment below describes an experiment in which which of the following is the dependent variable?

A new species of oceanic snail is uncovered by a biologist. By monitoring the development rate of the species as the water's temperature rose, he was able to determine whether it could withstand the heat. In order to assess which kind of marine habitat the snail would be most suitable for, he also examined two different salt concentrations.

a. **Growth rate**

b. Salt concentration

c. Temperature

d. Number of snails

49. Of the following, which one is a carbohydrate?

a. Myosin

b. Collagen

c. **Cellulose**

d. ATP

50. Which of the following areas of the neurological system is principally in charge of controlling all subconscious and involuntary muscle actions?

a. Peripheral nervous system

b. Autonomic nervous system

c. Somatic nervous system

d. **Sympathetic nervous system**

CHAPTER 4: English and Language Usage

You might be wondering, "Why is this on a nursing exam? As soon as your nursing profession formally starts, you'll have to communicate with a huge variety of patients, coworkers, and superiors regularly. You must have a solid foundation in the fundamentals of communication, which boils down to being able to write clearly and organize your thoughts. This will help you better understand how to react in the many scenarios that you'll face as a nurse and help you choose your words properly. On a more immediate note, throughout your nursing study, you will undoubtedly be required to write a considerable number of essays and other reports. Without the ability to communicate effectively, you cannot succeed or graduate.

To achieve a high score in the English and Language Usage section of the ATI TEAS test, you need to demonstrate a strong grasp of various language-related concepts. This section is designed to assess your understanding of grammar, sentence structure, punctuation, vocabulary, and the ability to effectively organize and improve paragraphs. Let's go through each aspect in detail:

1. Conventions and Standard English: This category evaluates your knowledge of standard English grammar and usage. You'll be tested on subject-verb agreement, pronoun usage, verb tense, adjectives, adverbs, and other grammatical elements. Make sure to review the rules of grammar, such as singular/plural forms, verb conjugations, and proper word order.

2. Punctuation: The punctuation section assesses your ability to use punctuation marks correctly. Topics may include periods, commas, semicolons, colons, apostrophes, quotation marks, and hyphens. Understand when and how to use each punctuation mark to convey clarity and meaning in a sentence.

3. Sentence Structure: This part focuses on sentence construction and syntax. You'll encounter questions related to sentence fragments, run-on sentences, sentence combining, and sentence rearrangement. Understanding how to create clear and well-structured sentences is crucial for this section.

4. Improving Paragraphs: In this segment, you'll be given a paragraph or passage with underlined portions that may contain errors or areas for improvement. You need to

identify the correct options for revising and improving the text. This requires a good understanding of grammar and coherence within a paragraph.

5. Vocabulary: Vocabulary questions gauge your knowledge of word meanings and context. Expect questions on synonyms, antonyms, analogies, and context-based word usage. Building a strong vocabulary through reading and studying word roots, prefixes, and suffixes can help you excel in this section.

6. How to Organize a Paragraph: This part assesses your ability to structure and organize a coherent paragraph. Questions may involve identifying topic sentences, supporting details, transitional words, and concluding sentences. Understand the flow of ideas within a paragraph to answer these questions effectively.

7. Knowledge of Language: The knowledge of language section delves into the broader aspects of language usage, including figurative language, idiomatic expressions, and rhetorical devices. Be familiar with various literary techniques and their meanings.

To succeed in the English and Language Usage section:

- Review grammar rules thoroughly, focusing on common errors and areas you may struggle with.

- Practice identifying and correcting punctuation errors in sentences and paragraphs.

- Work on building clear and concise sentences, avoiding sentence fragments and run-on sentences.

- Improve your vocabulary through regular reading and practice with synonyms and antonyms.

- Learn how to structure paragraphs effectively, with a clear topic sentence and supporting details.

- Familiarize yourself with literary devices and figurative language for the knowledge of language questions.

Remember, practice is key to improving your English and language usage skills. Consider using official ATI TEAS study materials, practice tests, and other reputable resources to prepare effectively for the exam. Good luck with your test preparation!

Questions & Answers

1. Which of the following is a correctly spelled word?

    A. Absence

    B. Absents

    C. Abcense

    D. Absense

Answer: Absence

2. Check to see if the highlighted part of the next sentence is accurate or if it needs to be changed. Sports are a significant part of life for people all across the world, as was demonstrated in 2006 when billions of people came together to be involved with the World Cup either through playing, watching or thru advertising.

    A. World Cup either through playing, watching or advertising

    B. World cup either through playing, watching or thru advertising

    C. World Cup either by playing, watching or through advertising

    D. World Cup either through playing, watching or thru advertising

Answer: World Cup either through playing, watching or advertising

3. Which of the following is a correctly spelled word?

    A. Restauratuer

    B. Presentor

    C. Photographer

    D. Dictatar

Answer: Photographer

4. Which of the following sentences best sums up the one below?

The letters were quite _____ and contained intimate details.

    A. Personal

    B. Personnel

    C. Personel

    D. Personal

Answer: Personal

5. Which of the following best describes the passage's genre?

    A. Look review

    B. Letter

    C. Fictional story

    D. Poetry

Answer: Poetry

6. Which phrase should go at the start of paragraph B to make the strongest impact?

    A. The TPS reports allow company stakeholders to monitor our productivity.

    B. Although the extended hours do represent a heavier workload, they regrettably do not boost creative production.

    C. This quarter, productivity rose in four departments.

    D. The November training schedule will put a strong emphasis on raising productivity.

Answer: This quarter, productivity rose in four departments.

7. To _____ should I address the postcard?

Which of the following accurately finishes the previous sentence?

    A. Who

    B. Whom

    C. Which

    D. The which

Answer: Whom

8. Which of the following articles is most likely to include these phrases?

    A. Stage play

    B. Business memo

    C. Scientific journal

    D. Poetry anthology

Answer: Stage play

9. Check to see if the highlighted part of the next sentence is accurate or if it needs to be changed.

Many high school students volunteer their time in the neighbourhood by working with their friends, young children, and senior persons.

    A. He volunteers his time to work with peers, young children, and senior residents in the community.

    B. They participate in community activities by working with classmates, young children, and senior residents.

    C. Participate in community activities by working with classmates, young children, and senior persons.

    D. They participate in community activities by helping their friends, small children, and senior residents.

Answer: They participate in community activities by helping their friends, small children, and senior residents.

10. Which statement is the most concise?

    A. I sent my parents off to boarding school when I was twelve years old.

    B. My parents sent me to boarding school when I was twelve.

    C. When I was twelve years old, my parents sent me to boarding school.

    D. My parents sent me to boarding school when I was twelve.

Answer: When I was twelve years old, my parents sent me to boarding school.

11. Which of the sentences below has a verb that agrees with the subject?

    A. The rescue group, which accepts animals from zoos around the nation, has consented to refrain from selling the elephants to another zoo.

    B. A reputable animal rescue group has received the remaining elephants.

    C. Only a few of the zoo's elephants have been given permission to transfer to the new habitat.

    D. The zoo's chief keeper, who has worked there for more than 20 years, has agreed to build the elephants a new habitat.

Answer: The rescue group, which accepts animals from zoos around the nation, has consented to refrain from selling the elephants to another zoo.

12. Which of the next statements from the passage is a complete sentence?

Kendra struggled to get any sleep the night before she departed for college. She was mulling over the potential outcomes of this journey. She questioned her potential roommate, her ability to get to all of her classes, and the extracurricular groups she might join. She was confident that the following chapter will bring her fresh and improved experiences.

    A. Which clubs she might join outside of school.

B. Kendra's final night before heading off to college.

C. She was confident that the following chapter will bring her fresh and improved experiences.

D. Could anticipate having fresh, improved experiences in the upcoming chapter.

Answer: She was confident that the following chapter will bring her fresh and improved experiences.

13. Which of these sentences, when included in a paragraph, is irrelevant?

    A. I used to sing "Circle of Life" by heart and perform for my folks in our living room.

    B. The third-longest running Broadway production and all-time top-grossing musical is The Lion King.

    C. I've wanted to be an actor since I was a young child, whereas some individuals may spend their entire lives searching for the ideal profession.

    D. When I was six years old, my mother took me to see The Lion King on Broadway, and I immediately felt at home there.

Answer: The third-longest running Broadway production and all-time top-grossing musical is The Lion King

14. Which of the following statements belongs in a research paper's citation list?

    A. According to the most recent World Health Organization report, asthma symptoms often worsen at night or after physical activity.

    B. Contrary to the World Health Organization's findings, which are discussed in section 2, this paper comes to the conclusion that asthma symptoms can be reduced with regular exercise.

    C. The current study investigates the connection between asthma and exercise.

    D. Wheezing, coughing, chest tightness, and shortness of breath are examples of asthma symptoms.

Answer: According to the most recent World Health Organization report, asthma symptoms often worsen at night or after physical activity

15. The following sentence's underlined portion needs to be changed:

Combining multiple devices with complementary features, such as a phone, music player, and planner's scheduling capabilities, is a growing trend in technology.

    A. The planner's scheduling capabilities.

    B. Additionally a planner with scheduling tools.

    C. Features for scheduling, too.

    D. A scheduler

Answer: A scheduler

16. Despite having a car, every morning _____ rides the bus to work.

    A. Car Michelle

    B. Car; Michelle

    C. Car, Michelle

    D. Car. Michelle

Answer: Car, Michelle

17. Dr. Jones had a _____ for speaking aloud, upsetting people frequently.

    A. Tendency

    B. Tendincy

    C. Tendancy

    D. Tendencie

Answer: Tendency

18. He was the model of ___, with exquisite taste and manners.

   A. Versatility
   B. Depravity
   C. Decorum
   D. Duplicity

Answer: Decorum

19. One of the hardest decisions for management is whether to fire a worker.

Which part of this statement needs to be revised?

   A. After "fire," add a comma.
   B. Conversion from managements to managements
   C. Substitute Weather for Whether.
   D. Managers should be changed to managers.

Answer: Conversion from managements to managements

20. Which word in the following statement is misspelt?

She was faced with a decision after receiving the invitation: should she attend the wedding or go out to dinner with her sister?

   A. Wedding
   B. Invitation
   C. Diner
   D. Dilemma

Answer: Diner

21. A chaperone is required to travel with the gymnasts when they go to a competition.

Which of the above statements best sums up the sentence?

    A. It

    B. Them

    C. All of it

    D. Their

Answer: Them

22. The audience was strongly _____ by the actors' performances.

Which of the following options accurately finishes the preceding sentence?

    A. Effected

    B. Affected

    C. Were effecting

    D. Were affecting

Answer: Were effecting

23. Which of the following approaches to revising and combining the highlighted text in the phrases below WOULD NOT be acceptable? Their primary benefit is a yearly pension payment. The amount of the pension has undergone numerous reviews and adjustments, most recently to reflect the pay of a senior government official.

    A. Pension payments each year; pension payout

    B. An annual pension payout; since 1958, the pension's amount has increased over time.

    C. A pension payout each year, the sum of which

    D. The amount of the pension payout made each year

Answer: Pension payments each year; pension payout

24. A post-mortem examination was carried out after contacting the medical examiner.

Which of the following words is a noun?

- A. Was
- B. Perform
- C. Medical
- D. Examination

Answer: Examination

25. The term underlined in the phrase below means which of the following?

Omari chose to leave his job and enrol in nursing school since he was disinterested in his work.

- A. Unsure
- B. Indifferent
- C. Dissatisfied
- D. Motivated

Answer: Indifferent

26. Our training enables you to get employment in a variety of fields, such as criminal justice and nursing information technology.

Which part of this statement needs to be revised?

- A. After breastfeeding, a comma should be used.
- B. After "job," add a comma.
- C. Following industries, omit the comma.
- D. After criminal, add a comma.

Answer: After breastfeeding, a comma should be used.

27. At Hudson University, most students look forward to their Chemistry classes.

Which part of this statement needs to be revised?

    A. After "University," add a comma.

    B. Substitute Chemistry for Chemistry.

    C. Rename the students to the pupils'.

    D. To Class, change class.

Answer: Substitute Chemistry for Chemistry.

28. The majority of businesses maintain precise estimates of their prophet margins and frequently demand attendance at weekly meetings. Which of the following Answer: s fixes the flaw in the previous sentence?

    A. There in place of there

    B. Change prophet to gain

    C. Attendance should be changed to Attendees

    D. Swap businesses for businesses'

Answer: Change prophet to gain

29. The annual _____ birthday party was thrown by Nichelle and Denise in Las Vegas.

    A. Her

    B. Their

    C. Theirs

    D. Hers

Answer: Their

30. You will be charged a late fee in the next two weeks if your payment is not received.

Which revision of this sentence would be most effective?

    A. You would be evaluated after two weeks.

    B. You were evaluated after two weeks.

    C. You were evaluated after two weeks.

    D. No revision is required.

Answer: No revision is required.

31. Which of the following phrases adheres to the capitalization rules?

    A. African white-backed vultures are dark-colored as young birds; their white feathers do not appear until they reach adulthood.

    B. The seasons on the planet Neptune continue for 41 Earth years because of its far from the sun.

    C. The first vaccine was created by Edward Jenner, who is known as the Father of Immunology.

    D. Men in costumes and masks play jokes on their neighbours during the Ukrainian festival known as Malanka.

Answer: Men in costumes and masks play jokes on their neighbours during the Ukrainian festival known as Malanka

32. Last weekend, _____ went to the movies.

    A. She and me

    B. Her and me

    C. She and I

    D. Her and I

Answer: She and I

80 | ATI TEAS

33. I'm going to _____ next year. Which of the following phrases best sums up the preceding sentence?

    A. I earned my college diploma.

    B. I've finished my college degree.

    C. I did earn a college degree.

    D. Will finish my college education.

Answer: Will finish my college education

34. He was the model of ___, with exquisite taste and manners.

    E. Versatility

    F. Depravity

    G. Decorum

    H. Duplicity

Answer: Decorum

35. Initial assessments of the damage to crops following the reactor meltdown were very challenging due to conflicting criteria for permissible radiation levels in foods.

    A. Conscious

    B. Intrusive

    C. Reliable

    D. Private

Answer: Reliable

36. Which comma completes the following sentence the BEST?

I have no idea how my book got to her place, but I do need it back.

A. .

B. ,

C. ;

D. :

Answer: ,

37. Which of these sentences is incorrect?

    A. If I'm not busy on Sundays, I relax on the couch and watch TV.

    B. If a student has a question, they should raise their hands.

    C. She placed the beach towel on the sand.

    D. Put the platter on the table, please.

Answer: Put the platter on the table, please.

38. After a while, _____, we were able to unlock the doors and exit the elevator.

Which of the following phrases best completes the previous sentence?

    A. In spite of

    B. Finally

    C. Before

    D. As an example

Answer: Before

CHAPTER 5: Reading

Benefits of reading:

Reading comprehension is an essential skill tested in the ATI TEAS (Test of Essential Academic Skills) exam. Here are some of the benefits of reading:

a. **Improves Comprehension:** Regular reading helps improve your ability to understand and interpret written information, which is crucial for success in the TEAS test.

b. **Enhances Vocabulary:** Reading exposes you to a wide range of words and phrases, expanding your vocabulary and improving your ability to grasp complex texts.

c. **Boosts Critical Thinking:** Reading involves analyzing and evaluating information. This skill is invaluable when tackling the critical thinking questions often found in the TEAS exam.

d. **Increases Retention:** Reading regularly strengthens your memory, helping you retain the information you need to succeed in the exam.

e. **Reduces Stress:** Reading can be a great stress-reliever, which is vital for managing test anxiety and maintaining focus during the TEAS exam.

Is reading really tiring?

The perception of reading as tiring can vary from person to person. Several factors can contribute to feeling tired while reading:

a. **Reading Level:** If the reading material is significantly above your current reading level, it may require more mental effort and concentration, leading to a feeling of fatigue.

b. **Reading Speed:** Slow readers might feel tired after prolonged reading sessions due to the increased time and effort it takes them to complete the same amount of content.

c. **Content Complexity:** Reading dense, technical, or unfamiliar subjects can be mentally taxing.

d. **Physical Comfort:** Reading for extended periods in uncomfortable positions or environments can lead to physical fatigue.

However, regular practice can improve reading stamina, and choosing engaging and suitable material can make reading less tiring over time.

Technology and reading

Technology has significantly impacted the way we read, and this has implications for preparing for the TEAS exam:

a. **Digital Texts:** Many TEAS test-takers may find themselves reading digital texts during the exam. It's essential to practice reading from screens to become comfortable with this format.

b. **Online Resources:** Technology has made it easier to access various reading materials and practice questions relevant to the TEAS exam. Utilize online resources to supplement your preparation.

c. **Interactive Learning:** Some test prep platforms offer interactive reading exercises that simulate real exam scenarios. These can be valuable in improving comprehension and retention.

d. **Distractions and Focus:** While technology offers convenience, it can also be distracting. Practice maintaining focus during digital reading sessions to avoid losing valuable study time.

Preparing for the exam

Effective preparation for the ATI TEAS test involves targeted reading practice and other strategies:

a. **Study Materials:** Obtain study guides and practice books specifically designed for the TEAS exam. These will familiarize you with the test format and types of questions.

b. **Practice Reading Tests:** Regularly take full-length practice tests to assess your reading comprehension skills and identify areas that need improvement.

c. **Time Management:** Work on your reading speed and comprehension to manage time effectively during the exam.

d. **Annotate and Summarize:** Practice annotating and summarizing passages to improve understanding and retention.

e. **Diverse Reading Material:** Read a variety of texts, including science articles, social studies passages, and technical material, to prepare for the diverse topics in the exam.

f. **Consistency:** Set aside dedicated time for reading practice daily to build stamina and improve skills gradually.

g. **Test-Taking Strategies:** Familiarize yourself with test-taking strategies, such as skimming passages before reading questions or eliminating answer choices to increase accuracy.

Test Simulation 1

Systolic blood pressure categories are listed in the table below.

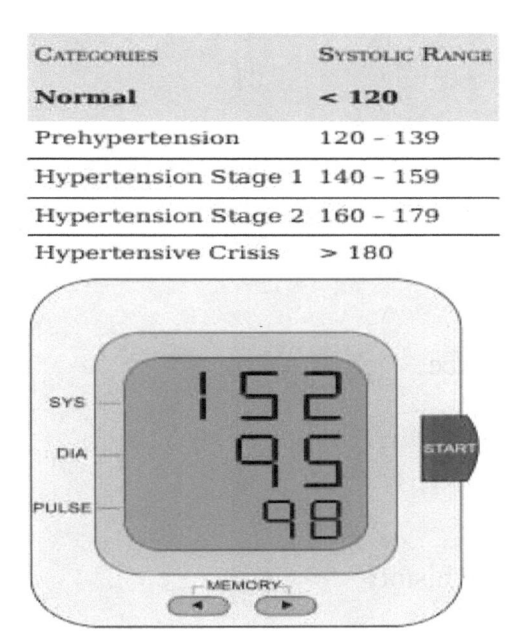

Categories	Systolic Range
Normal	**< 120**
Prehypertension	120 – 139
Hypertension Stage 1	140 – 159
Hypertension Stage 2	160 – 179
Hypertensive Crisis	> 180

SYS 152
DIA 95
PULSE 98

The blood pressure reading for a patient is seen above.

1. What classification does the patient fit into?

    a. Normal

    b. Normal

    c. Stage 1 hypertension

    d. Stage 2 hypertension

Answer: Stage 1 hypertension

The following table forms the basis for the following three questions. A classification scheme for libraries is the dewey decimal system.

Dewey decimal classification

000 works in information, computer science, and other fields

101 psychology and philosophy

Religion 200

Social sciences 300

400 languages

500 in both science and math

600 applied and technical science

700 arts and leisure

Literature 800

900 biography, geography, and history

2. Teddy has been given the task of writing a history essay about the us during the cold war. Noam chomsky is an american linguist, philosopher, social scientist, cognitive scientist, historian, social critic, and political activist. His teacher suggested that he read some of chomsky's writings. Teddy checked the dewey decimal classifications since he wasn't sure where to start. What combination of the following three classes, while not exhaustive, would probably be the most useful?

A. 100, 300, 700

B. 100, 300, 800

C. 100, 400, 900

D. 200, 300, 900

Answer: 100, 400, 900

3. Teddy developed an interest in post-world war ii anarchism, a social science theory that asserts the political philosophy that rejects a coercive government, while researching chomsky's numerous theories and arguments. The best works on the topic are what he is looking for. Which area of the library has the greatest chance of having the necessary books?

A. 000

B. 200

C. 300

D. 900

Answer: 300

4. Teddy wants to explore traditional judaism as it was practised in the early 20th century after learning about chomsky's jewish origins during his investigation. Which area of the library is most likely to provide the information you need?

A. 100

B. 200

C. 300

D. 900

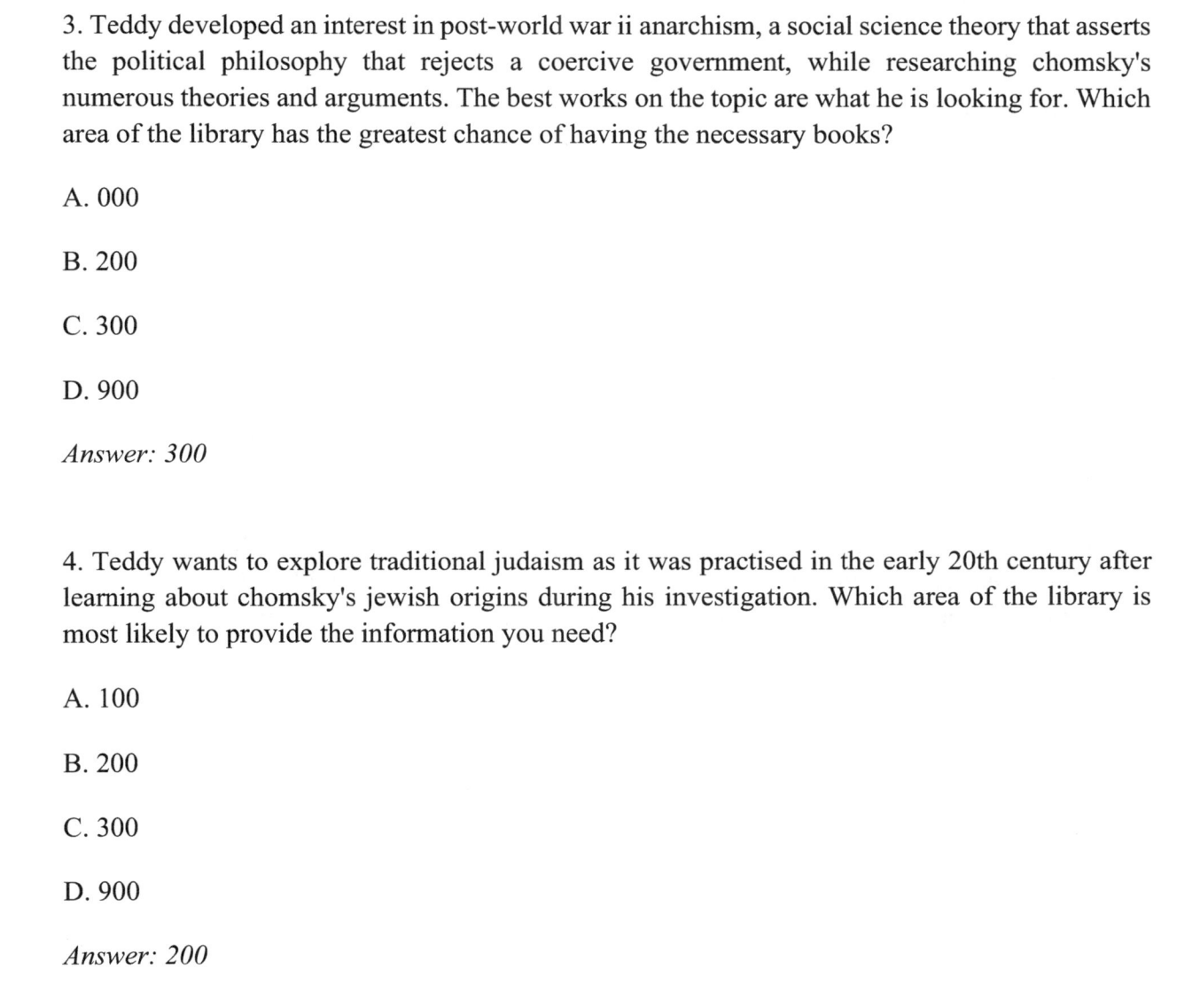

Answer: 200

The section from which the next question is based.

America's social and political discourse is still heavily infused with idealism. According to an idealistic perspective, americans must keep striving for the truths of freedom, equality, justice, and human dignity. Truth, according to idealists, is what ought to be, not necessarily what is. They strive to make things better and as close to perfect as they can.

5. Which of the following sums up the author's intention the best?

    A. To promote liberty, justice, equality, and human rights

    B. To describe an idealist's worldview

    C. To discuss why social and political discourse in america is flawed

    D. To persuade readers to accept particular facts as true

Answer: To describe an idealist's worldview

The section from which the next question is based.

In one of the largest cities in the united states, samuel is a high school teacher. His students come from a variety of family types. Samuel notices that the top pupils in his class come from homes with little parental oversight. By far the most involved parents are those of the bottom five students. His class consists of 24 pupils. Based on the academic success and familial backgrounds of his students, samuel will compose an academic article. The study will make the case that parental involvement is not a significant determinant of academic achievement.

6. Which of the above phrases accurately sums up samuel's sample size?

    A. The sample is skewed because he is familiar with the individuals personally and has firsthand experience with them.

    B. There aren't enough participants in the sample to draw conclusions that apply to a sizable group.

    C. There are too many participants in the sample to comprehend the particulars and context of each student's circumstance.

    D. The sample is impartial and the right size to make inferences about the importance of parental supervision in education.

Answer: There aren't enough participants in the sample to draw conclusions that apply to a sizable group.

On this passage, the following four questions are built.

In the world of snakes, skin tone and markings are very significant. The creatures can conceal from predators thanks to the intricate swirls, diamonds, and stripes, but probably most significantly (for us humans, at least), the patterns can also reveal whether a snake is dangerous. Even though it may seem illogical for a poisonous snake to stand out in brilliant red or blue, that elaborate outfit signals to any nearby predator that it would be unwise to approach him.

However, just because a snake has striking patterns doesn't imply it will be dangerous; certain snakes have developed defence mechanisms that work without venom. The deadly coral snake, with which the scarlet kingsnake frequently coexists in the same habitat, bears extremely similar patterns to the scarlet kingsnake. The kingsnake, however, is not venomous; it is only acting poisonous to humans. Because a hawk or eagle that hunts predationally from a great height cannot detect the difference between the two species, the kingsnake is passed over and survives to fight another day.

7. Why did the author decide to write this essay in the first place?

    A. To clarify how a snake's poisonous status relates to its markings.

    B. To help readers understand the distinction between kingsnakes and coral snakes.

    C. To show how poisonous snakes are.

    D. To show how animals adapt to harsh conditions and survive.

Answer: To clarify how a snake's poisonous status relates to its markings.

8. What can be inferred from the passage above by the reader?

    A. The kingsnake poses a threat to people.

    B. The same predators hunt both the coral snake and the kingsnake.

    C. Because it's simple to determine whether a snake is toxic, handling them in the woods is safe.

    D. When hawks or eagles are nearby, the kingsnake's markings alter.

Answer: Because it's simple to determine whether a snake is toxic, handling them in the woods is safe.

9. What is the best summary of this passage?

   A. Humans can tell whether a snake is poisonous by its hue and markings.

   B. Animals often employ colouring to conceal from predators.

   C. The coral snake and scarlet kingsnake have almost identical patterns.

   D. Bright markings are a common feature of venomous snakes, however nonvenomous snakes can also imitate those hues.

Answer: Bright markings are a common feature of venomous snakes, however nonvenomous snakes can also imitate those hues.

10. Which of the following best describes the passage's goal?

   A. To educate

   B. To amuse.

   C. To explain

   D. To influence

Answer: To educate

The passage that the following question is based on is.

Annabelle rice began to have problems falling asleep. She developed a nocturnal schedule as a result of an abrupt malfunction in her biological clock. She initially believed her insomnia was a result of staying up late writing a horror story, but she later realised it was actually because she was so terrified of the bright outside world. She came to the conclusion that she now had heliophobia.

11. Which of the following best captures the significance of the underlined word in the previous sentence?

   A. Aversion to dreaming

   B. Aversion to sunlight

C. Aversion to strangers

D. Spectrum of anxiety disorders

Answer: Aversion to sunlight

Read the passage that follows. Then respond to the query.

Today, numerous shark species are listed as endangered. The main cause of this is human activity. Sharks are targeted by fishing industries due to their commercial and cultural relevance. Traditional chinese medicine prize shark fins as a component. In asia, shark fin soup is regarded as a delicacy. Each year, 100 million sharks are killed as a result of the practise of "shark finning," which involves catching sharks, cutting off their fins, and dumping the carcass.

12. What would be the finest addition to this passage?

　　A. When pursuing tuna, fishermen occasionally unintentionally catch other species in their nets.

　　B. There is an increasing market for shark fins in hong kong and elsewhere, making them just as lucrative as other fish.

　　C. Environmental organisations are focusing more on overfishing on a global scale.

　　D. Every other year, mothers of sharks give birth to one litter of eight to twelve young.

Answer: There is an increasing market for shark fins in hong kong and elsewhere, making them just as lucrative as other fish.

Read the instructions that follow. Then respond to the query.

1. Begin your sentence with users kid.

2. Reverse the word sequence.

3. Place the letter n before the second word's first vowel and after the first vowel in the first word.

4. Reposition the fifth letter of the second word such that it comes after the word's first vowel.

13. Which words have you formed?

    A. Kin ruses

    B. Dnk nurses

    C. Ink ruses

    D. Kind nurses

Answer: Kind nurses

On this passage, the following two questions are founded.

Before planting, learn how to plant potatoes.

Potatoes should be planted no later than two weeks following the final spring frost.

One to two days prior to sowing, chop potatoes into pieces.

Use a hand trowel or a tiller to loosen the soil. Incorporate compost or fertiliser into the loosening soil.

Planting

Potatoes should be placed 4 inches deep and 4 inches apart.

Cover potatoes loosely with dirt.

Following planting

After planting, water the area immediately and then frequently to keep the soil moist.

After six weeks, build up dirt around the plant's base to keep the roots protected.

14. Which of the following should be done as the first thing after planting potatoes?

    A. Pile earth up around the plant's base.

    B. Drink water right away.

C. Combine compost or fertiliser with the loosening soil.

D. Set your potato spacing at one foot.

Answer: Drink water right away.

Q15: after a tiller or trowel has been used to remove the soil, what should be done next?

A. Combine compost or fertiliser with the loosening dirt.

B. Create a trench 4 inches deep.

C. Slice up some potatoes.

D. Pile earth up around the plant's base.

Answer: Combine compost or fertiliser with the loosening dirt.

Read the nutrition information on the accompanying label. Then respond to the following two questions.

Nutrition Facts

Serving Size (343g)
Servings Per Container

Amount Per Serving

Calories 310   Calories from Fat 60

	% Daily Value*
Total Fat 6g	9%
Saturated Fat 1g	5%
Trans Fat 0g	
Cholesterol 0mg	0%
Sodium 70mg	3%
Total Carbohydrate 58g	19%
Dietary Fiber 7g	28%
Sugars 23g	
Protein 5g	

| Vitamin A 15% | • | Vitamin C 6% |
| Calcium 30% | • | Iron 15% |

*Percent Daily Values are based on a 2,000 calorie diet. Your daily values may be higher or lower depending on your calorie needs:

	Calories:	2,000	2,500
Total Fat	Less than	65g	80g
Saturated Fat	Less than	20g	25g
Cholesterol	Less than	300mg	300mg
Sodium	Less than	2,400mg	2,400mg
Total Carbohydrate		300g	375g
Dietary Fiber		25g	30g

Calories per gram:
Fat 9 • Carbohydrate 4 • Protein 4

16. A high-calorie, low-fat diet has been recommended for an underweight patient by the doctor. If this cereal makes up a third of his diet, is it appropriate?

    A. No, the cereal has too many calories and fat.

    B. No, the cereal does not have enough calories but is appropriately low in fat.

    C. The cereal is adequately rich in calories and low in fat, so the answer is yes.

    D. The cereal is appropriately low in calories and high in fat, so the answer is yes.

Answer: No, the cereal does not have enough calories but is appropriately low in fat.

17. The doctor advises the patient, who has diabetes, to consume no more than 200 g of carbohydrates every day. Does the patient who consumes three meals each day find this cereal to be a good choice?

    A. The 58 g of carbohydrates are less than one-third of the 200 g total, so the answer is yes.

    B. The 58 g of carbohydrates are fewer than the daily limit of 200 g, hence the answer is yes.

    C. No, as the 58 g of carbohydrates make up more than a third of the entire 200 g.

    D. No, because 58 grammes of carbs per day is considerably too little for someone with diabetes.

Answer: The 58 g of carbohydrates are less than one-third of the 200 g total, so the answer is yes.

The following passage serves as the basis for the next four questions.

Smoking is awful.

Tobacco use has terrible negative effects. A single cigarette contains nearly 4,000 compounds, including 43 recognised carcinogens and 400 lethal poisons. Tar, carbon monoxide, formaldehyde, ammonia, arsenic, and ddt are a few of the more hazardous components. Numerous cancers, including those of the throat, mouth, nasal cavity, oesophagus, stomach, pancreas, kidney, bladder, and cervix, can be brought on by smoking.

Nicotine, one of the most addicting drugs ever created, is found in cigarettes. The definition of addiction is a compulsive need to seek out the substance despite repercussions. Nearly 35 million smokers reported a wish to stop smoking in 2015, according to the national institute on drug abuse, yet more than 85% of those addicts will not succeed in their endeavour. Most smokers regret lighting up their very first cigarette. If you have not yet begun smoking, it would be prudent for you to take note of their error.

Nearly nine million americans suffer from a significant smoking-related ailment, and 16 million americans now have a smoking-related condition, according to the u.s. Department of health and human services. The centers for disease control and prevention (cdc) estimate that tobacco use results in close to six million deaths annually. By 2030, this number is anticipated to increase to over eight million deaths. On average, smokers pass away ten years sooner than nonsmokers.

In the us, tobacco products are often taxed by the municipal, state, and federal governments, which raises their cost. Some smokers spend more money on a pack of smokes than they do on a few tanks of petrol. Smokers also frequently smell. The stench of smoke fills the air and gives off an overpowering unpleasantness. Smokers run the additional risk of developing yellow tar residue stains on their teeth and fingers.

Smoking is dangerous, expensive, and unattractive to others. Smoking clearly isn't worth the hazards.

18. Which of the following statements best sums up the passage?

    A. Storytelling
    B. Convincing
    C. Expository
    D. Technical

Answer: Convincing

19. Which of the following summaries of the passage, is most accurate?

    A. Compared to many alternatives, tobacco is less healthier.
    B. Smokers would be much better off giving up the habit because tobacco is dangerous, expensive, and socially unappealing.
    C. Tobacco products are frequently taxed by local, state, and federal governments in the united states, which raises their cost.
    D. Tobacco products cause more than six million deaths annually and cut smokers' lives short by ten years.

Answer: Smokers would be much better off giving up the habit because tobacco is dangerous, expensive, and socially unappealing.

20. Which of the following claims would the author be most likely to agree with?

    A. Smokers should abstain from using any nicotine replacement therapies and only quit cold turkey.

    B. Substances other than tobacco are more addictive.

    C. Smokers should give up for whatever motivation leads them to do so.

    D. Those who want to keep smoking should push for lower taxation on tobacco products.

Answer: Smokers should give up for whatever motivation leads them to do so.

21. Which of the following answers indicates an author opinion statement?

    A. According to the centers for disease control and prevention (cdc), tobacco products cause almost six million deaths per year.

    B. People who are dependent on nicotine may spend more on a pack of cigarettes than on a few gallons of gas.

    C. They also run the risk of getting tar residue on their fingers and teeth.

    D. Smokers also often smell bad. The stench of smoke fills the air and gives off an overpowering unpleasantness.

Answer: Smokers also often smell bad. The stench of smoke fills the air and gives off an overpowering unpleasantness.

The next two questions are based on this map.

22. Of the following, which is directly north of the fire circle?

   A. A mature oak tree

   B. Scouting camp

   C. Pond with fishing

   D. Outdoor camping

Answer: Scouting camp

Q23. Which of the following would a camper have to pass through if she took the trail from the fishing pond to the scout camp and passed the fire circle on her way?

   A. Vintage oak tree

   B. Station ranger

   C. Backcountry camping

   D. Pier

Answer: Vintage oak tree

Examine the passage. Answer the query after that.

According to law enforcement officials, texting and driving is becoming more common among teenagers in the us. In spite of being aware of the risks, 35% of teen drivers admitted to texting and driving in a aaa survey. In the united states, one out of every four car accidents is the result of texting while driving. Teenage girls are undoubtedly to blame for the majority of these collisions because they appear careless and rarely pay attention while driving. Young drivers in particular should put their phones away while operating a vehicle. About eleven teenagers die every day as a result of texting and driving, according to aaa.

24. Which of the following statements from the passage best captures the author's viewpoint?

    A. According to law enforcement authorities, teens in the us are increasingly texting and driving.
    B. Teenage girls are undoubtedly to blame for the majority of these collisions; they exhibit a lack of caution and attention while driving.
    C. Despite being aware of the dangers, 35% of teen drivers admitted to texting and driving in a aaa survey.
    D. According to aaa, texting while driving claims the lives of about eleven teenagers every day.

Answer: Teenage girls are undoubtedly to blame for the majority of these collisions; they exhibit a lack of caution and attention while driving.

25. Which of the following would serve as the article's primary source for the battle of gettysburg?

    A. A letter from a local farmer who saw the conflict
    B. A local tv station's documentary about the conflict
    C. A war novelization written by a union soldier's great-grandson.
    D. A history book used in a college-level american history course.

Answer: A letter from a local farmer who saw the conflict

The passage from which the following five questions are based.

For julia, the morning had been exhausting. The sound of lawnmowers outside her window had woken her up early, and despite her best efforts, she had been unable to fall back asleep. She reluctantly made her way out of bed, took a shower, and made her coffee for the day. She at least made an effort. She had realised in the kitchen that she was out of regular coffee and had to settle for a cup that was decaffeinated.

Her caffeine-free coffee didn't make the unpleasant traffic any less annoying once she got on the road. It actually took julia an extra fifteen minutes to get to work since she thought the other drivers were just as slow and grumpy. Additionally, every parking space was taken when she arrived.

By the time she'd finally located a spot in the overflow lot, she was thirty minutes late for work. She had assumed that her boss would be too busy to notice, but he had already placed a stack of documents on her desk with the message, "rewrite." she debated whether or not to inform her supervisor that the reports hadn't actually been written by her, but she ultimately opted against it.

An hour later, when the fire alarm went off, julia had had enough. Along with her coworkers, she gathered her purse and went outside. While everyone else waited for the alarm to stop, julia marched resolutely to her car, started the motor, and headed for home.

26. Which of the following is the most likely reason julia did not return to work after the alarm?

      A. She felt humiliated that she couldn't complete the task her supervisor had assigned.

      B. She wanted to go home since she was exhausted.

      C. She was unable to return to her office because of a traffic jam.

      D. Her boss granted her a day off.

Answer: She wanted to go home since she was exhausted.

27. According to the passage, which of the following statements should be regarded as an opinion?

      A. Julia's manager requested that she complete some work for one of her coworkers.

      B. Julia arrived at work late due to traffic.

C. It was irresponsible for julia to leave work early.

D. Julia had been woken up early, so she was exhausted.

Answer: It was irresponsible for julia to leave work early.

28. Which of the following accurately outlines julia's activities in order?

    A. Julia got up early and noticed she didn't have any ordinary coffee. Her boss had a lot on her plate when she arrived at work. She made the decision to return home after the fire alarm sounded.

    B. When julia arrived at work, she realised she was too exhausted to complete the tasks her boss had assigned, so she left to get a cup of coffee at home.

    C. When the fire alarm went off, julia was awakened and was unable to go back to sleep. She then got caught in traffic and was 30 minutes late for work.

    D. A lawnmower woke julia up early, and on the way to her office, she got caught in traffic. She arrived to discover that the office was short on coffee and that she had a tonne of work to do. She made the decision to return home after the fire alarm sounded.

Answer: Julia got up early and noticed she didn't have any ordinary coffee. Her boss had a lot on her plate when she arrived at work. She made the decision to return home after the fire alarm sounded.

29. Julia set a course for home, according to the passage's last sentence. Which of the following statements best describes how this sentence should be understood?

    A. Julia can't return home right away.
    B. Julia intends to travel by car.
    C. Julia will return to work even though she wants to go home.
    D. Julia is concerned that the fire at her workplace will spread to her residence.

Answer: Julia intends to travel by car.

30. Which of the following conclusions does the passage support the strongest?

A. A job nearer julia's house will be found for her.

B. Julia will lose her job.

C. Julia will feel bad and go back to work.

D. Julia will drive home and then retire to bed.

Answer: Julia will drive home and then retire to bed.

A brief introduction to the subject is followed by the following five questions, which are based on the chart.

1861 to 1865 saw the fighting of the american civil war. The only civil war in american history was this one. While the south's secession served as the war's catalyst, other factors such as slavery and divergent views on the rights of individual states also contributed to the conflict. Robert e. The general

Throughout the war, lee commanded the confederate army for the south. Ulysses s. Grant ended the war as the successful general despite the north using a variety of lead generals. The civil war saw more american deaths than any other military conflict in american history.

Civil War Casualties by Battle (approximate)					
Battle	Date	Union General	Confederate General	Union Casualties	Confederate Casualties
Gettysburg	July 1863	George Meade	Robert E. Lee	23,049	28,063
Chancellorsville	May 1863	Joseph Hooker	Robert E. Lee	17,304	13,460
Shiloh	April 1862	Ulysses S. Grant	Albert Sydney Johnston	13,047	10,669
Cold Harbor	May 1864	Ulysses S. Grant	Robert E. Lee	12,737	4,595
Atlanta	July 1864	William T. Sherman	John Bell Hood	3,722	5,500

31. Which of the following battles saw more confederate deaths than union deaths?

    A. Cold harbor

    B. Chancellorsville

    C. Atlanta

    D. Shiloh

Answer: Atlanta

32. Which of the ensuing battles took place first?

    A. Cold harbor

    B. Chancellorsville

    C. Atlanta

    D. Shiloh

Answer: Shiloh

33. Which of the following engagements did robert e. Lee not command the confederate soldiers in?

    A. Atlanta

    B. Chancellorsville

    C. Cold harbor

    D. Gettysburg

Answer: Atlanta

34. Which of the following battles saw the largest disparity between union and confederate casualties?

    A. Cold harbor

    B. Chancellorsville

C. Atlanta

D. Shiloh

Answer: Cold harbor

35. Which of the following conflicts saw more than twice as many american casualties as the overall number of casualties in the battle of gettysburg?

    A. Cold harbor

    B. Chancellorsville

    C. Atlant

    D. Shiloh

Answer: Shiloh

After a brief introduction to the subject, the next two questions are based on the accompanying visual.

In order to determine the population and demographics of the country, the united states constitution commands congress to conduct a census of the population. The survey is conducted by the united states census bureau. The first u.s. Census was carried out in 1790 by thomas jefferson, who was then secretary of state. The most recent census was carried out in 2010. The following census in the united states will be the first to be conducted primarily online.

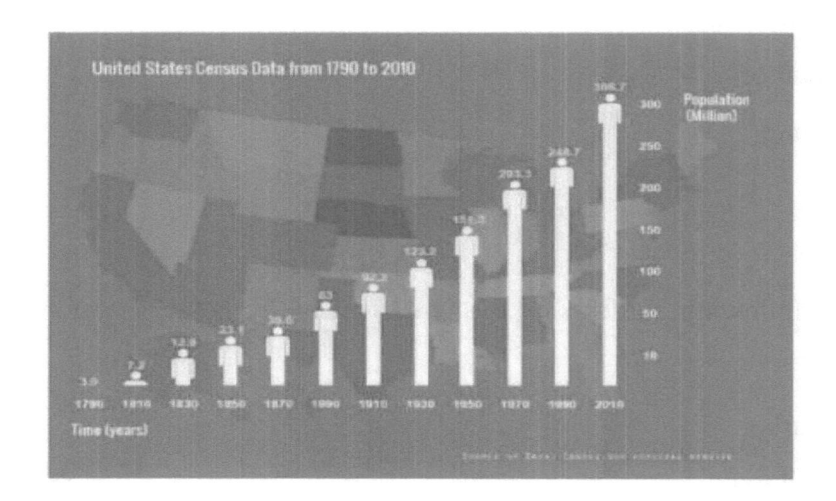

36. Which of the following years saw fewer people living in the united states than in 1930?

    A. 1950

    B. 1970

    C. 1910

    D. 1990

Answer: 1910

37. What year saw the largest population growth over a twenty-year period?

    A. Between 1930 and 1950

    B. Between 1950 and 1970

    C. Between 1970 and 1990

    D. Between 1990 and 2010

Answer: Between 1990 and 2010

Check out the passage. Then respond to the following query.

Not because marie didn't like the new student at her high school. With her friendly demeanour and easy grin, lucinda graham got along with practically everyone. The issue developed when lucinda started to surpass marie in her customary skills. For instance, after joining the softball team, lucinda quickly took marie's place as the leadoff batter and shortstop. The first games marie had ever lost at school were in the chess club when lucinda made marie resign three times in a row. There were now rumours that lucinda's science project would be selected as the institution's sole submission in the state science fair, the same event where marie had won first place the year before. In a month, the election for class president would take place. Marie, the popular incumbent, at least had that as a backup.

38. Which of the following predictions about this narrative would you make?

    A. Marie will opt not to seek the position of class president.

B. Marie's opponent in the race to be class president is lucinda.

C. Marie and lucinda will collaborate to support a different candidate for class president.

D. Lucinda would brag about her triumphs over marie and fall out of favour with the pupils.

Answer: Marie's opponent in the race to be class president is lucinda.

Check out the passage. Then respond to the following query.

In the short story the old man and the sea by ernest hemingway, an elderly cuban fisherman has tried day after day for eighty-four days without success. The other fishermen make fun of him because of his mistakes. The young apprentice's parents ban him from going with the elderly man any more since they believe he is unfortunate. After a two-day, arduous battle, the old guy finally hooks a massive marlin on the 85th day and reels it in. He returns home after lashing the marlin to his boat. Sharks attack his tiny boat, consume the marlin, and only the skeleton is left. The elderly guy successfully docks his boat before stumbling off to seek some rest. A group of fisherman are astounded to see the marlin's eighteen-foot skeleton still clinging to the boat the following day. They understand how much effort the elderly man put into catching and bringing in the fish. The young apprentice of the old man offers to go with him on his next expedition.

39. Which of the following best encapsulates the main idea of this tale?

    A. Despondency of old age

    B. The challenge of marlin fishing

    C. Age against youth

    D. Tenacity and bravery

Answer: Tenacity and bravery

The following query is based on this passage.

Chapter 2: texas amphibians

Frogs

A) Tree frogs

B) -------

C) Genuine frogs

Toads

A) True toads

B) Narrowmouth toads

C) Toads that burrow

Salamanders

40. Which of the following is a logical heading to insert in the empty space, according to the pattern in the headings?

A) Gray tree frog

B) Frogs from the tropics

C) Newts

D) Spadefoot toads

Answer: Frogs from the tropics

Read the author's justification. Then respond to the following query.

The moment has arrived for female marathon runners to participate in international competition with male runners.

41. Which of the following statements contradicts the above argument?

A) More women than ever before are participating in weekend 5k and 10k races, according to data collected around the nation.

B) Winning times for women in major marathons around the world are decreasing faster than winning times for men, according to runner's world magazine.

C) A current sports medicine specialist points out that since running is an endurance-based sport rather than one that depends on raw strength or speed, women may be better suited to compete against males in this sport.

D) A well-known worldwide running coach claimed this year in an interview that with the right preparation, women may soon compete favorably with men in marathons and other long-distance events.

Answer: More women than ever before are participating in weekend 5k and 10k races, according to data collected around the nation.

Read the text. Then respond to the query.

1960's presidential election

A theological issue

Former republican vice president richard m. Nixon ran against democratic senator john f. Kennedy in the 1960 presidential election. The contest was dominated by foreign policy and rivalry with the soviet union during the cold war. However, the campaign also raised issues related to religion. Because kennedy was a roman catholic, some nixon backers contended that he would have been more devoted to the pope than to the u.s. Constitution. Although nixon officially gave his team the order not to bring up the subject during the campaign, the dispute persisted all the way through november.

Initially broadcast debate

The first presidential debate on television included kennedy and nixon. The two contenders sparred about current affairs, including as the economy, the alleged missile gap with russia, and the newly installed communist government in cuba. Both sides had compelling arguments during the discussion. Strangely, the decision seemed to be determined by the television cameras. In contrast to those who watched on television, people who heard the discussion on the radio believed that nixon had won. Nixon talked with authority but perspired a lot in the harsh studio lights, making him appear anxious and hopeless. Kennedy won the day because to his slick demeanor in front of the camera. Every american election, according to historian theodore h. White, "calls upon the individual voter to balance the past against the future." * for american voters, kennedy looked to represent the future. He prevailed in a tight race for the president.

42. Why is the footnote in this paragraph important?

    A) To clarify the second paragraph's subject

    B) To clarify how religion came to be a contentious topic in the 1960 presidential election

    C) Cite the quote's author in the second paragraph.

    D) To provide more details regarding the 1960 election

Answer: Cite the quote's author in the second paragraph.

After a brief introduction to the subject, the next three questions are based on the image.

Biologists utilize a food chain diagram to clarify how ecosystems work. It symbolizes the interactions between various animals and plants. Through photosynthesis, plants transform the energy from the sun into stored energy that moves up the food chain. When a creature dies and decomposes back into the earth, energy is returned to the ecosystem. This procedure is a never-ending circle.

Living things are categorized into main producers and consumers, which have several layers, in food chains. For instance, tertiary consumers eat primary consumers while secondary consumers eat primary consumers. Animals at the top of the food chain are known as apex predators. Apex predators are the highest category of consumers in an ecosystem, and they lack natural predators.

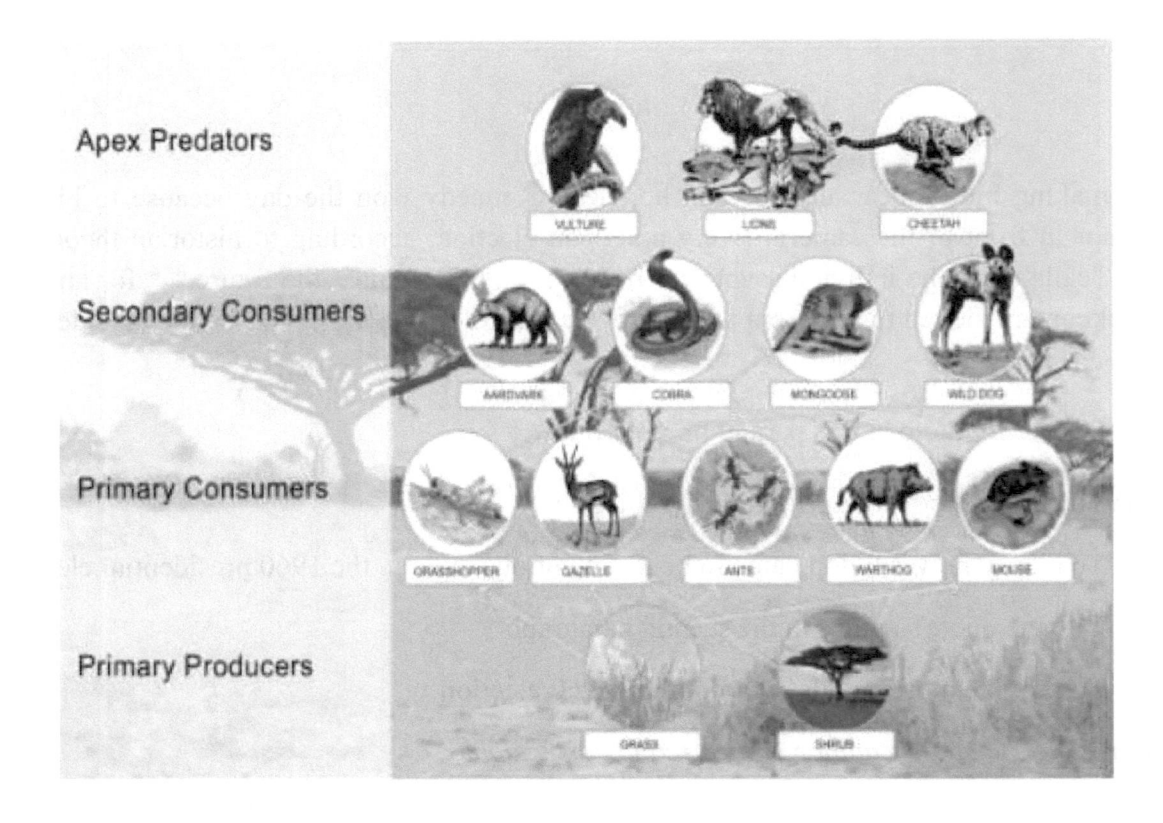

Apex Predators: VULTURE, LIONS, CHEETAH

Secondary Consumers: AARDVARK, COBRA, MONGOOSE, WILD DOG

Primary Consumers: GRASSHOPPER, GAZELLE, ANTE, WARTHOG, MOUSE

Primary Producers: GRASS, SHRUB

43. Which of the following species, according the food chain diagram, consumes primary producers?

   A) Snake

   B) Gazelle

   C) A wolf

   D) Aardvark

Answer: Gazelle

44. Which of the following species, according to the food chain diagram, has no natural predators?

   A) The vulture

B) Snake

C) Mongoose

D) Aardvark

Answer: The vulture

45. Which of the following would a mongoose consume, question number six?

A) Grass

B) Aardvark

C) Vulture

D) Mouse

Answer: Mouse

Test Simulation 2

CONCLUSION

Having gone through this book, you have encountered many practice questions that have given you a taste of what to expect on the ATI TEAS. We hope that you have been able to understand the different question types and the content of the questions. We have tried to actually give detailed explanations for the many question types. The test covers the basics of academic skills that you acquire while studying in high school. However, there are even more detailed materials that you should study.

Additionally, it is vital that you have time to rest during your week. You should give yourself the opportunity to do something fun and meaningful for a few days in your week. All work and no rest is going to burn you out, and your grades and test score may suffer. Finding time for yourself is also important. So you should try to find the opportunities to exercise, do self-care, go to the park, and socialize with friends. At the same time, you should actually bear in mind your goal and the fact that you want to go to nursing school. You must guard your time and your schedule and effectively craft your study plan.

This book is not the magic book that will provide all the answers. Rather, we want it to be a resource that will lead you to find the answer if you have any questions or concerns. We consider this book to be a large but not exhaustive resource. Given our efforts to research the answers to your questions, we hope that you have been able to understand how to study for the exam. Our detailed answer explanations provide you with the needed teachings from the test. These explanations come from experience with the material, as well as research that has been conducted to find the answers. We urge you to continue your search for all the answers. Study hard. Practice will enable you to achieve great things. Know that you are on a great path. Becoming a nurse is an honorable and sacrificial path that is rewarding and enjoyable, but it takes a lot of hard work. We hope you will realize this as you are preparing for the ATI TEAS. But once you have given the hard work and dedication, you will not look back. A life of diligence will become your mantra. You will work long and hard, but you will do it for the benefit of humanity. The world needs more nurses to take care of the sick and elderly. And this is just the beginning—the beginning of a wonderful and meaningful career.